The DON'T DIET, LIVE-IT! Workbook®

Healing Food, Weight and Body Issues

By
Andrea Wachter, LMFT
Marsea Marcus, LMFT

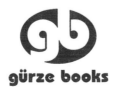
gürze books

The Don't Diet, Live-It!® Workbook
Healing Food, Weight and Body Issues

Copyright © 1999 Andrea Wachter and Marsea Marcus

Published by:
Gürze Books
PO Box 2238
Carlsbad, CA 92018
(760)434-7533
www.gurze.com

Cover design by Abacus Graphics, Oceanside, CA
Cover image copyright ©PhotoDisc, Inc.; selected by Patricia Andersson

ISBN 0-936077-33-6

NOTE:
The authors and publisher of this book intend for this publication to provide accurate information. It is sold with the understanding that it is meant to complement, not substitute for, professional medical and/or psychological services.

The following are trademarks of InnerSolutions: Live-It® and InnerSolutions™
The authors can be contacted at: InnerSolutions; 5905 Soquel Dr. #650; Soquel, CA 95073; (831) 476-7500; www.innersolutions.net; info@innersolutions.net.

All client names are pseudonyms to protect confidentiality.

We use the pronoun "she" throughout this book and hope that men reading it will translate where necessary to make the information applicable.

This book is dedicated to ending food obsession and body hatred.

In loving memory of:
Jack Marcus
Evelyn Grand
Ida and Jack Wachter
Adele and Julius Steinhauer
and Neil

Acknowledgments

Marsea and Andrea would like to thank:

- Santa Cruz O.A., without which this book would not be possible.

- Dr. Bob and Bill W. for pioneering the path to recovery and Rozanne for making it available to compulsive eaters.

- Geneen Roth, Carol Munter and Jane Hirschmann for pioneering the non-diet approach.

- Stephanie Brown, an inspirational author and theorist who developed the stages of recovery for alcoholics. We used her stages as a model for people with food, weight and body issues.

- All of the courageous clients in our groups for testing out these Journeys with their lives.

- Laura Golden Bellotti and Deborah Abbott for their wonderful editing and cheerleading.

- Anya Abrams and Joel Primack for generously giving us our first computer.

- Carol Inez Charney for her creative ads and graphic design for InnerSolutions.

- Jennifer Chase for the many projects and errands she did for us, and advance thanks for many more to come!

- Nancy Bazor for helping us get organized.

- Eric Schoeck for his diligent and thorough help proofreading the manuscript.

- Joan Barnes-Strauss for finding us and believing in us.

- Jewish Family and Children's Services of San Francisco for giving us another forum for our ideas.

- Process Therapy Institute for their brilliant techniques and instruction.

- Leigh Cohn and Lindsey Hall Cohn of Gürze Books for their impeccable timing in finding us and for taking this book on its next Journey.

Marsea would like to thank:

- All the people who loved and supported me when I could not love or support myself: Mom, Dad, Chris Parks, Miriam Goldberg, Morgen Alwell-Bartel, Juli Vinik, Erica Golden, Ellie Freedman, Gail Faris, Barbara Marcus, Lynette Marcus, Diana Grand, Sam Grand, the women of My Kin Talk, Bill Marcus, Stephen Grand and Andrea.

- *And the man who found me when I could:* Jamie F. Amos.

- Also, my honorary homies: Ken Bewick and Cynthia Strauss for being wonderful people.

Andrea would like to thank:

- An incredible group of friends and mentors who daily show me the way on my Journey.

- My mom for her gift of empathy, my dad for his sense of humor and my whole family for their endless generosity, love and encouragement.

- Marsea for many things, not the least of which is typing the entire book on her computer and never once complaining when I delivered chapters and ideas on little yellow Post-its!

- Neil Brown, Stefanie Elkin and Robyn Wesley for, in their own unique ways, teaching me how to be a therapist.

- Pam Gruen for her brilliant marketing skills and for always believing in me.

Contents

INTRODUCTION ix

CHAPTER ONE: Outer Solutions vs. Inner Solutions 15

CHAPTER TWO: Isolation vs. Reaching Out 28

CHAPTER THREE: Thoughts vs. Feelings 40

CHAPTER FOUR: Stuffing vs. Acknowledging Feelings 54

CHAPTER FIVE: Aggressive vs. Assertive Communication 67

CHAPTER SIX: Criticism vs. Praise 81

CHAPTER SEVEN: Black-and-White vs. Rainbow Thinking 97

CHAPTER EIGHT: The Binge/Deprive Cycle vs. Loving Limits 111

CHAPTER NINE: Emotional vs. Physical Hunger 131

CHAPTER TEN: Diet vs. Live-It 146

CHAPTER ELEVEN: Weight Control vs. Natural Weight 161

CHAPTER TWELVE: Competition vs. Camaraderie 177

CHAPTER THIRTEEN: Holding On vs. Letting Go 193

CHAPTER FOURTEEN: Human Doing vs. Human Being 206

CHAPTER FIFTEEN: Endings vs. Beginnings 219

Appendix A: National Non-Profit Organizations 238

Appendix B: Support Groups 240

Appendix C: Websites 241

Appendix D: Recommended Reading & Tapes 242

Appendix E: For Professionals — Leading Live-It® Groups 245

Introduction

As licensed counselors, with many years of experience leading groups and helping individual clients with food, weight, and body issues, we've long had an interest in creating a book to help others. At least as important as our professional credentials is the fact that we've both "been there" with food, weight, and body issues of our own.

Having spent most of our lives in the grips of dieting, overeating, sneaking food, being fat and miserable, being thin and miserable (and being every weight in between), we each embarked on a Journey of Recovery. We use the word "Journey" here because we have found that recovery is a process, a Journey. It is not a single event, a destination, or a number on the scale. It is a way to live. The process involves changes, challenges, and insights. Much like traveling to any unknown location, it can be scary. The only reason that we were both willing to go on this Journey was that we had each come to a point in our lives where we knew we were at a dead end; our food compulsions, self-hatred and body obsessions had us trapped in a prison that had become intolerable.

We discovered that the first necessity on our respective Journeys was to break our isolation. We each had thought we were the only ones who struggled so intensely with food and weight issues. There were no maps or directions on boxes of cookies or bags of chips to tell us where to go for help. And there was no one to guide us after our latest diet ended or failed. Fortunately, we were each led, separately, to a support group where we learned to be honest about our feelings, our eating and our lives. When we began to admit our problems to, and share our pain with, people in the group, we learned that we were not the only ones who suffered in this way. We discovered there were other people who had found or created maps with directions to guide them, and later us, on the Journey of Recovery.

Next we learned that hating ourselves hindered rather than helped us in this process. We had always thought that if we could just get to the "perfect" weight, we would like ourselves and be happy. **We now know that no weight is ever perfect enough to do the enormous job of creating happiness.** We found that we had to first accomplish the difficult tasks of liking ourselves and treating ourselves well before we could ever live comfortably in our bodies.

The next leg of our Journey has been a long one (in fact, we're still on it!). Instead of focusing on where we are going and whether or not we will ever arrive (and how many calories, or lost pounds it will take to get there), we now focus on the trip itself. We notice who is traveling with us, and we are aware of and curious about the surrounding scenery. We found that focusing on food and weight kept us from seeing and being in the moment, and from knowing what we really needed. We had to teach ourselves to pay attention while driving, to travel at our own pace, to stop when necessary, honk the horn when in danger, and to get regular tune-ups along the way. In other words, we had to learn how to be present, how to take care of ourselves in the moment, and how to cope with problems that arise. Yes, it got rocky at times, and sometimes we even got lost or broken down; but we, and hundreds of our clients, found this Journey incomparably more rewarding than that old trip from the couch to the refrigerator, to the scale and back again.

We think it's important that you know a little bit about who we are and how our separate Journeys began.

Andrea:

I spent most of my life hating my body, obsessed with food, and starting and failing countless diets. As a teen, I dieted with friends and family members, and snuck food after meals. However, as the years progressed, and the pain that fed my eating continued to go unchecked, so too did my insane relationship with food and my body.

By the time I started college, I had gained and lost the same 30 lbs. so many times that (as Lily Tomlin once said) "my cellulite had déjà vu." I did not know the source of my pain because all my attention was focused on my weight and the food I ate. I became bulimic (although I had not even heard of the term then). What began as an innocent experiment in weight control turned into an eight-year addiction to bingeing and purging. At one point, I realized I was out of control and could not stop. What now strikes me so deeply about that period is that I had so many friends and family members around me, and yet nobody knew of my silent agony.

Each day I courageously tried to "start fresh," "be good," eat just a little. Each evening, however, after finally breaking down and stuffing myself with food, I ended up full of remorse and self-hatred. Vomiting as an attempt to get rid of the food and feelings only made me feel worse. These were extremely painful years. My sickness around food, and disgust with my body, colored every area of my life. Because of my low self-esteem, I felt inferior to other women and had unhealthy interactions with men. I was always uncomfortable in my clothing, and I had difficulty focusing on my studies because, although I ate a lot, I was undernourished. I was also unclear about what I was going through.

*It was Geneen Roth's first book, **Feeding the Hungry Heart**, that finally proved to me that somebody else (actually, lots of somebody elses) felt out of control with food and weight. Realizing for the first time in my life that I was not alone was the most liberating feeling I had ever experienced. This revelation led me to seek therapy and a support group. I began to learn about the emotional pain inherent in my binges, the unexpressed anger in my vomiting, and the deep grief hidden within my excess weight.*

It has been a long, hard, and wonderful road since then. This Journey is what this book is about. I have succeeded in recovering from bulimia and body perfectionism, and now I am committed to helping others do the same.

It's hard to believe that my greatest pain has led me to my greatest joys: a wonderful career, self-love, and intimate, loving relationships in which I can fully be myself. I could never have dreamed of so much during my days alone on the couch with food as my closest friend.

Marsea:

Part of me will always be amazed that I actually recovered from what was once a life of bingeing, dieting, bingeing, hating myself, and more bingeing.

When I was 17 years old I wrote in my diary, "I have to eat nothing or else I eat everything; that's just the way it is." Around that time I turned fasting into an art form, starving myself for weeks at a time in order to "reduce the damages" from my binge-eating. I also became an expert on nutrition and health foods so that I could eat "perfectly" in front of others and keep my secret life with food a secret. The way I ate in public prompted people to tell me, "You have such amazing willpower!" or "I could never discipline myself like you do!" They only saw me eating salads and vegetables, never eating boxes of cookies, gallons of ice cream, or all the leftovers from the plates in the kitchen.

Years later, at the height of my food addiction, I could no longer even pretend I had willpower. I was 60 lbs. above my most comfortable weight, living alone in the mountains (in an attempt to get away from food) and unable to work. It seemed to me that every job involved food, looking good, or the ability to concentrate, and I was so out of control I couldn't even consider trying. I felt like I was on the outside of society, looking in: my whole world was about my eating and my weight, while other people seemed to have actual lives they were living.

Recovery hasn't been easy, yet it has become one of my greatest accomplishments. I am no longer obsessed or out of control with food. In fact, food and I have a friendly, peaceful, and sometimes distant relationship. I have achieved the weight loss I had always dreamed of, but the process was slower and deeper than expected. And it had very little to do with what I ate! (Quite different from the quick and easy, short-term fix with which diet clubs enticed me.) I now have a body I like, a life I enjoy (much of the time), and a self that is good to me and fun to be around.

Our Journeys have taught us how to better navigate life's challenges, exit roads we didn't want to be on, and head in the direction of health and freedom. We learned that when we stuffed our painful feelings down, positive feelings got stuffed as well. Recovery was not only about finding our pain. It was also about finding our joy, our creativity and our heart's desires. We now live with full lives rather than full stomachs. Our latest adventure, creating this workbook, has been another fulfilling road trip. We invite you to join us.

How to Use This Workbook

This book is designed to combine the personal and creative aspects of a journal with the more structured and guided aspects of a workbook. Each of the 15 chapters focuses on an essential aspect of recovery and includes an explanation, personal stories and a series of questions or exercises. The Journey One questions are for your first time through the book. We recommend that you date each entry so that on later Journeys you can reflect back on your previous travels.

After you've completed your first Journey through the book, you are ready to begin Journey Two. To do this, reread each chapter, then complete the Journey Two exercises that follow it. It is important to reread each chapter, because during each reading you will have a new perspective of your Journey and, as a result, you will have new understandings. We've included four different Journeys, but feel free to take as many trips as you like by photocopying pages or inserting blanks. Much like regular drives along your favorite scenic route, each trip is a different and unique experience. We hope you will take several excursions through your workbook. Reviewing your progress, as well as obstacles, is valuable and helpful along the road to recovery.

Periodically, throughout your workbook, you will come across the following sign:

This sign designates what we call a *Spontaneous Road Trip*. A Spontaneous Road Trip is akin to deciding to go off the beaten path and explore unknown territory. This sign will be followed by a blank page upon which we encourage you to do whatever you want. You can use it to express anything that's going on for you at the time you come across it. Draw or write spontaneously about your thoughts and feelings, make a collage, write a poem, insert a photograph of yourself . . . anything you can come up with as a way to explore and record the current part of your Journey.

We encourage you to treat yourself gently on this Journey. We have found for ourselves that compassion is an essential element of the healing process. You wouldn't be here now if you weren't already suffering. Can you acknowledge this by showing some compassion for yourself? After all, if you came upon a child who had been badly hurt, would you be rough and critical with her, or kind and loving? We recommend you cultivate an empathetic attitude toward yourself. It may be difficult, especially after many years of overeating, depriving yourself, and hating your body. But we ask you: How has your negative thinking and self-hatred helped you so far? If beating yourself up was helpful in your quest to lose weight, you most certainly would be thin and happy by now. **Nothing positive comes from treating yourself negatively!** So how about trying another way?

Travel Tips

TRAVEL AT YOUR OWN PACE. You can answer one question a week or one topic a week. You can spend a month on each section, or complete an entire Journey in a weekend. There is no right or wrong way to do this book. If certain questions don't apply to you or don't seem helpful, skip them. This is *your* Journey, and *you* are the navigator.

BE SPONTANEOUS. Usually the first thing that comes to mind is significant, so try to write it down before your critic arrives to censor you. There are no right or wrong answers, and you are not being graded, so be as honest as you can.

KEEP YOUR BELONGINGS IN A SAFE PLACE. Just as it's safer to leave your luggage in the trunk of the car rather than in the back seat where it can be seen, we recommend that you find a private place to keep your workbook. Do whatever is necessary to insure that this very personal belonging is not violated. The safer you feel, the more honest you can be.

DON'T TRAVEL ALONE IN DANGEROUS TERRITORY. In the course of writing, there may be times when feelings come up that are scary or embarrassing. Usually a strong reaction means that you are on the threshold of a new discovery about yourself. Oftentimes, this is when people quit writing and/or turn to food. We strongly suggest that, instead, you find safe people with whom you can share your threatening or fearful feelings.

Some examples of safe people are:
- a supportive friend
- a psychotherapist
- a support or self-help group
- a close, loving family member

We wish you a safe and loving trip filled with many new discoveries! Don't Diet, Live-It!

Chapter One

Outer Solutions vs. Inner Solutions

All we see of other people are their outsides. We see their faces and their bodies, their clothes, houses, and cars. That's also what other people see of us. Sometimes we believe that this is all there is. However, we each have an inner world that is far more important than what we show and see on the outside.

Most of us haven't been taught how to show our true feelings to others. We may have tried as children and found that they weren't welcomed or well-received. No matter how loving, caring, or available our parents may have been, they could not possibly have met all our needs. Sometimes our parents can't figure out what we need because our own needs are very different from what they needed when they were children. And sometimes our parents are unable to give us what we need because they didn't get their own needs met. It takes a lot of conscious work and commitment to change the legacy of hurt and unmet needs that may have been passed down in our families for generations.

Many of us found solace in food when we could not find it in our families. Food was something we could count on. Everything else was unstable — parents might disapprove or be critical, friends might tease or turn on you, your best efforts might not result in success or happiness. But ice-cream is *always* creamy, peanut butter is *always* rich, and chocolate is *always* sweet.

Food can be a solution for some things. It can end hunger, give nourishment, and provide pleasure. **But there is no food that can combat loneliness, anger, shame, sadness, or anxiety.** These are inner issues that need inner solutions. When we become obsessed with food and our bodies, we are trying to solve inner problems with outer solutions.

Marsea:

> *When I was fat, my goal in life was to become thin. This goal consumed
> 15 crucial years of my life, from the time I was 15 until I was about 30. I tried
> numerous diets, "food plans," exercise programs, and health-oriented theories.*

But every attempt ended in failure. Why? Because I never addressed the reasons I was numbing myself with food. I thought my only problem was that I was fat. I thought that my fat caused me to be lonely and prevented people from being attracted to me. I would look around and imagine that the thin women had all the boyfriends.

While I know it is true that many people are fat-phobic and judgemental, I also know, now, that there are many large people who have no problem attracting friends and lovers. I look around me now and I notice people of all sizes who have love in their lives. And I see what I failed to notice before: there are thin people who are deeply unhappy and have unsatisfying relationships. Happiness is not related to body size! I came to realize the problem was not my fat, the problem was my thinking! My problem wasn't my weight, it was how I lived and that I used food to cope with problems.

Searching (as I did) in the diet industry for an answer to my "weight" problem was, therefore, unlikely to be helpful. It was not until I realized that my body was not the problem, that I started to make the internal changes that ultimately led me to permanent changes in my eating habits and, subsequently, my weight. I had to look inside, at myself, not outside at a diet. I had to become acquainted with my inner self, the part of me that held my unexpressed emotions, my unresolved problems, and my unhealed pain. I did not know this part of myself. I did not know I had years of angry, sad and hurt feelings inside of me, stored up from past events. I honestly thought that my only problem was my weight, and that if I could be thin, all would be well.

A therapist suggested that I write out my life history. I wrote what I thought was a wonderful story of all the fun and exciting things I had done. I painted a picture of a life that was great, except for one unbearable problem: my weight. Somehow, I forgot to mention my parents' divorce, the teacher who sexually harassed me, the traumatic surgery I had when I was 16, the therapist I struggled to trust who later betrayed me, my drug abuse, and the numerous unwanted and unpleasant sexual encounters I had experienced. I had spent several years in therapy focusing on my weight and my eating, and I had never mentioned any of this! I was an expert on nutrition, exercise, calories, and dieting, but I was completely ignorant about who I really was.

After writing my initial life history and seeing how incomplete and one-sided it was, I became determined to explore the reality of my life and get to know my inner self. That was when my recovery truly began. I wrote a second life history, and I told the truth.

Early on in the recovery process, many people have no idea who they really are and what their truth is. Not only have they used food and other outer distractions to silence themselves and hide their true feelings; they have also spent much of their time focusing on other people's feelings and needs. Of course, there is nothing wrong with caring or being concerned about other people. However, if it is at your own expense, it is not only unhealthy for you, it is likely unhealthy for the person for whom you are sacrificing yourself.

Many of our clients see themselves as "chameleons," adapting to the likes and dislikes of the people around them. Most of them fear that their needs or feelings will upset or anger other people. Being uncomfortable with their own feelings, they are also unable to tolerate anybody else's feelings. There is a difference between focusing on and trying to "fix" other people's feelings and actually being able to tolerate and accept their feelings. As you become familiar with your own needs and feelings, you will learn how to be comfortable with other people's feelings as well.

As long as you are focused on outer solutions—"fixing" other people, buying a new car, having a thin body, having a baby, falling in love, earning more money—you will not be able to address the inner pain that drives you away from yourself in the first place. The process of recovery leads you inward to learn who you really are and what you really need.

The recovery process can be seen as having four distinct stages: *Denial, Transition, Early Recovery*, and *Ongoing Recovery*. In each stage you will have different challenges and needs, and a different relationship with food and your body.

The *Denial Stage* is when we still believe that if only we could be thin, or control our eating, everything would be okay. We think that lack of "willpower" is our problem (when in fact many of us have exhibited extraordinary "willpower"). We continue going on diets, despite the fact that they have always failed us in the past. We keep thinking this next diet is going to do it, and if we just lost weight, we will finally be happy. We deny the fact that there is an emotional component to our eating problems, and we tend to keep our feelings and problems to ourselves. Our emphasis in this stage is on outer solutions.

In the *Transition Stage* we realize that our problems go deeper than the size of our bodies. We become more aware of what triggers our self-destructive eating patterns and body obsessions. While we continue struggling with food, weight and/or body image, we have begun to accept that we need to look toward inner solutions, rather than outer solutions. We begin to accept that our problems have to do with our unresolved inner feelings and our insufficient ways of coping with life. These are not simple issues that can be fixed by a diet. At some point in the Transition Stage we start letting go of our self-destructive behaviors, such as bingeing, purging, or food deprivation, though we do not do it all at once. Consequently, we begin to experience the emotions we were previously avoiding. At this point, we often enter a crisis period, as we have not yet learned coping skills for our emotions. On top of that, many of us have *years* of suppressed emotions, and the emergence of these feelings can be a very difficult and frightening experience. Therefore, in this stage, a person requires an enormous amount of emotional support. Reaching out for help can be excruciatingly difficult, but without adequate support, the emotions are too overwhelming and cause many people to return to the Denial Stage (i.e. bingeing or dieting). How to create and utilize the type of support this stage requires will be discussed throughout this book.

Once our support system is in place and we are using it as needed, we enter *Early Recovery* and things start to calm down. While in the Transition Stage we needed to rely strongly on our support system, in Early Recovery we begin to be able to depend on ourselves a little more. When we do need help, we find it easier to reach out. We also develop an increased tolerance for handling our emotions, and we begin to get better at coping with them. In this stage, we do a lot of experimenting to discover what works for us and what doesn't in terms of our eating. As we see real changes happening within, we begin to have faith in the recovery process. This faith is especially helpful if we have not yet reached our natural body weight, which often doesn't occur until the next stage.

Ongoing Recovery is an ongoing process. It is about knowing and trusting ourselves and treating ourselves with love and respect. We become more and more comfortable with food and our bodies, and we know the steps to take when we experience difficult feelings. We are better able to identify our needs and speak our truth. We still use our support system, but support is less crisis-oriented and more a healthy choice. We have honest and intimate relationships, many that we developed in the course of our recovery, and it is natural for us to reach out to them for help when we need it. It does not mean we are perfect people, perfect eaters or perfect at anything. It means that we now know how to deal with life in a nonaddictive, conscious, mature and honest manner.

You may recognize yourself in one or more of these stages. Although we have been generalizing here to give you an idea of the itinerary for your Journey, recovery is a very individual and personal process. There is no way to do it other than your own way, and there is no appropriate pace at which to travel other than your own pace. You are your own tour guide on this Journey, responsible for where you go and with whom you travel. We are your travel agents, showing you the various options.

You may be just beginning your Journey, or you may be further along the continuum. Wherever you are at this juncture, we invite you to take a turn inward. The writing exercises in this book will help you learn to focus on your internal experience. It may take some time for you to get to know your inner self, just as it takes time to get to know another person. By the same token, the more time you spend with your inner self, the more you'll get to know that part of you. Becoming involved in your workbook is a way to introduce yourself to your deeper self, to spend time with that part of you, and ultimately better understand yourself and your hungers.

❧ *Journey One*

Date: _____

1. What are some external things (outer solutions) you think would make you happy? (i.e. losing 10 pounds, having a baby, getting a new job)

_____

_____

_____

_____

2. Add to the *Inner Pain* list some problems with which you are struggling. Add to the *Outer Solutions* list the ways you attempt to solve them.

Now, drawing lines, match up the inner pain with all the outer solutions you use to deal with it.

Inner Pain	Outer Solutions
feeling fat (insecure)	dieting
self-hatred	excessive exercising
feeling hopeless	throwing up
unresolved anger	buying new clothes

3. What feelings came up as a result of doing this?

_____

_____

_____

4. List one time when you felt like a "chameleon" this week (adapting yourself to fit in with others, rather than remaining genuinely yourself):

_____

_____

_____

_____

5. Write about what you think would have happened if you had acted authentically in the above situation?

_____

_____

_____

_____

6. What stage of recovery do you think you are presently in and why? (See pg.17)

_____

_____

_____

_____

7. What are some things you can do to focus on your *inner* self rather than your *outer* self?

_____

_____

_____

_____

CONGRATULATIONS! You have just completed your first Journey! (Remember, Journeys Two, Three, and Four are for subsequent trips through the workbook.) Now, continue Journey One by skipping ahead to Chapter 2.

❧ *Journey Two*

*Date:*_____

1. Referring back to Journey One, Question #1, which *outer solutions* did you attain (if any)?

_____

_____

_____

_____

2. Did obtaining these things make you happy? For how long?

_____

_____

_____

_____

3. Now write a list of the current "outer solutions" you think will make you happy:

_____

_____

_____

_____

_____

_____

4. Notice what you have omitted from, or added to, the list since Journey One.

5. List three recent situations when you put other people's needs ahead of your own, even though doing so *did not* feel right to you:

_____

_____

_____

_____

6. List three recent situations where you put someone else's needs ahead of your own and doing so *did* feel like the right thing to do:

_____

_____

_____

_____

_____

_____

7. At what stage of recovery do you currently think you are? (See pg. 17)

_____

This sign designates what we will call a *Spontaneous Road Trip*. A Spontaneous Road Trip is akin to deciding to go off the beaten path and explore unknown territory. When you arrive at this sign in your workbook, we encourage you to do whatever you want on this page. You can use it to express anything that's going on for you at this time. You can draw, write spontaneously about your thoughts and feelings, make a collage, write a poem, insert a photograph of yourself... anything that will help you explore and record this current part of your Journey. (Remember, there is no right or wrong way to do this!)

❧ *Journey Three*

*Date:*_____

1. Make a list of things you think would make you happy.

_____

_____

_____

_____

_____

_____

2. Which things on your list are obtained internally? Which things are obtained externally?

_____

_____

_____

_____

_____

_____

3. Identify the feelings that are connected to wanting each thing on your list.

Example: I feel sad, uncomfortable, and ashamed that I'm not at my ideal weight.

_____

_____

_____

_____

_____

_____

4. What do you think would truly be comforting to you when you're having those feelings?

Example: Someone just listening to me and not trying to fix me.

_____

_____

_____

_____

_____

_____

5. What stops you from doing/receiving the above actions?

_____

_____

_____

_____

_____

_____

6. What are the pros and cons of your food and weight issues?

_____

_____

_____

_____

_____

7. What stage of recovery do you think you are presently in, and why?

_____

_____

_____

_____

❧ *Journey Four*

*Date:*_____

1. List three personal experiences that have taught you that outer solutions are temporary and do not heal or satisfy you.

_____

_____

_____

_____

_____

2. List three personal experiences that have illustrated to you the healing power of addressing your internal needs.

_____

_____

_____

_____

_____

3. Draw a picture of yourself when you are avoiding your internal needs. (No artistic talent necessary, it can be realistic or abstract.)

4. Draw a picture of yourself after you have connected with someone and gotten your emotional needs met (even if just briefly).

5. What feelings were you aware of while drawing the above pictures?

_____

_____

_____

_____

6. What is one "inner solution" that you are needing right now?

_____

_____

_____

_____

_____

7. Are you willing to get that for yourself? Why or why not?

_____

_____

_____

_____

_____

Chapter Two

Isolation vs. Reaching Out

Although most addictions have some element of secrecy, food addictions and obsessions tend to be more hidden than most. Addicts and alcoholics have gathering places (bars, concerts, parties) where they socialize while engaging in their addictions. There is a feeling of camaraderie between them, even though it is rooted in the denial of their self-destructive behavior. Although food addicts do overeat (or undereat) in public, most food-related behaviors, like sneak-eating, bingeing, frequent checking of weight, vomiting, and examining oneself in the mirror (to name just a few) are done alone. Whereas alcoholics often get noticed for their drunken behavior, rambling speech, irresponsibility, or trouble with the law, the food-obsessed person often goes unnoticed. Many people with food and weight issues are experts at appearing strong, "together," and problem-free. Even if weight gain is noticeable, rarely is it mentioned, due to the negative images, fears, and taboos our society has regarding weight gain.

Bulimics have often been called "The Silent Screamers," anorexics are said to be "starving for attention," and binge eaters are described as "hiding behind a wall of fat." The commonality of all three? Each feels completely alone. And this makes sense. How do people foster intimate, loving, and authentic relationships with others when their deepest, most intense relationship is with food?

Although their struggle with food and weight was the biggest issue in their lives, many of our clients said that they hid it even from those closest to them. Husbands never knew of the years they spent throwing up in the bathroom after every meal. Best friends often had no idea they were suicidal over their weight. Children were unaware that nighttime binges were the reason Mommy was in such a bad mood in the morning.

At the core of food, weight, and body issues is a deep well of shame. Shame is what you feel when you believe that you are a failure as a person or that something is fundamentally wrong with you. When you feel shame, there is a tendency to isolate yourself (or your true feelings) from others. You may believe that you don't deserve support, so you keep your problems to yourself. Or you think your pain will "bring people down" so you hide it where others won't see it. The more secretive you become, the more alone you feel. The more alone you feel, the more your feelings of shame seem confirmed.

The good news and the bad news here seem to be one and the same. The good news is you don't have to be alone on your Journey of Recovery. The (seemingly) bad news is you can't recover alone. This is probably not what you want to hear; going on yet another diet might seem easier than having to include other people in your healing. If other people felt safe to us, we would not have turned to food to meet our emotional needs in the first place.

Since reaching out to others is essential to recovery, it is important that the people you reach out to are *Safe people*. Safe people are those who respect you and are good listeners. They do not try to fix you. Safe people welcome you and all your feelings, no matter what your feelings happen to be at the time. When you are done talking to a safe person, you feel heard and cared about. Safe people also know how to take care of their own feelings. When they need support, you can trust that they will find someone (whether it is you or someone else) who will listen and help them get their needs met. Safe people will also tell you when they can't be there for you. Although this may be difficult for you to hear, you will be able to trust that when they tell you they can be there, they really mean it.

Unsafe people are those who do any of the following: criticize, interrupt, try to "fix" you, respond dishonestly, give unsolicited advice, relate everything you say to themselves, or reveal your confidences. Usually, people turn to unsafe, rather than safe, people due to a fear of intimacy. We continue to go to unsafe people because their rejection and criticism, though painful, is familiar. Though many of us desperately crave compassion and understanding, the honesty and intimacy involved can be terrifyingly unfamiliar.

Different people can meet your needs in different ways. For example, a safe counselor (or psychotherapist) has special training and objectivity and can give you professional guidance on difficult or sensitive issues. A safe support group member may personally relate to your struggles and have similar experiences to share. A safe friend may be there for you on a more regular basis, for longer periods of time. A safe family member may have a special understanding of your history and a deeper, more unconditional love than anyone else. And someone ahead of you on your Journey may play a special role as a mentor—someone you can turn to for direction, hope and honest reassurance.

Reaching out to safe people means being honest. It means calling them or being with them when you are in pain or feeling bad about yourself. It means telling the truth when you are angry or hurt. It means asking for help when you don't know what to do. It means trusting people who are trustworthy.

Andrea:

It is still astounding to me that after so many years of sneak-eating and bingeing and purging in complete isolation and secrecy, I now talk openly about my issues with food. For years, not one soul knew how much pain I was in. Today I know that secrecy was a big part of my problem.

When my bulimia was discovered, I was encouraged to get help by attending a local support group for bulimics and compulsive eaters. One night, after the group, a woman came up to me and handed me her telephone number on a piece of paper. She said, "My name is Sally, and I want you to know that you can call me anytime." I can't recall what polite thing I said, but I remember thinking, "Yeah—right—in a million years!" Still, I put the paper in my coat pocket and went off to my private life of eating and purging and hating myself.

Some time later, I was driving home from work, and taking one of my regular detours to a little food mart in a nearby town. As I approached the store, filled with the insatiable, ravenous hunger that preceded a binge, I remembered that I had this woman's phone number in my pocket. Something had begun to change in me since attending that support group. I was beginning to understand that I was not the only person who did such crazy things with food, and that it probably wasn't all about food. I must be having feelings! I had thought that the only feeling I ever had was "fat." But the group members had said that "fat" wasn't a feeling — it was a body sensation and a judgment.

I saw the pay phone outside the store, and I'll never forget the dilemma I experienced. I thought, "What will I say?. . .I don't want to bother her. . . She didn't really mean what she said. . .She's probably not home anyway." I even picked up the phone and hung it up a few times before finally dialing. In order to get myself to make the call, I told myself I could eat after I made the call, if I still wanted to. I finally dialed, and when Sally answered the phone I said, "This is Andrea and you said I could call." She responded, "I'm so glad you did! What's going on?"

That call was my first connection to another person who could truly understand my feelings when I couldn't. I can't remember much of the conversation, except that at some point I realized I no longer needed to binge and, indeed, I made it home that night without bingeing. I got what I was really hungry for — human connection. This is not to say that I never binged again, but thanks to Sally and my own courage, I didn't binge that night. I started to see the value in reaching out to others. The phone calls got easier. I kept waiting for someone to say "What do you want?" or "Just don't eat" or "It's no big deal," but no one did. I called (and I still call) people who will understand. I call people who have been where I am or who are where I want to go. Breaking my isolation has had a profound effect on my recovery.

As you can see, it is very important to find safe people you can use for support on your Journey. One reason for this is what we call the *Same Brain Theory*. This theory states that the same brain that has developed into the unhealthy thinking patterns that lead you to overeat (or undereat) and obsess about your body, cannot suddenly think in a new and healthy way.

Your unhealthy patterns have taken many years to evolve, and you will need to hear and be reminded of the principles of recovery many times before these new ways become automatic. You need to hear about recovery from people who have been there, people who can listen to and tolerate your painful emotions and give you helpful suggestions for getting through them.

Most likely, this will not be a family member, even if your family loves you and is well-intentioned. Loved ones usually want you to feel better right away. They don't understand that it's important to fully experience your feelings. They may say things like, "Oh, don't let it get you down," or they may try to help by getting into premature problem-solving. What they may not be able to do is welcome your painful feelings and encourage you to express them. For this reason, it is often better to turn to uninvolved or objective, safe people.

Safe people can help you get through difficult events and situations without compulsively overeating. They do this by listening to you, loving you unconditionally, and encouraging your honest expression of feelings. One way to utilize your safe people is a technique called *Bookending*. Bookending is when you call a safe person prior to a difficult situation, talk about your situation, receive support, and then call back again after the situation is over.

One of our clients, Rachel, has a very difficult time after talking to her mother on the telephone. Her mother is critical of her weight; she shames and belittles her. When she gets off the phone, Rachel feels ashamed and worthless. In the past she turned to food, and ended up hating herself even more. Since Rachel has decided that she wants to stay in contact with her mother, but is also aware that she is not yet able to stand up to her, we suggested bookending these phone calls. Now Rachel calls group members before and after calling her mother. As a result of having someone safe to express her feelings to, Rachel no longer turns to food after speaking with her mother. And because her safe people remind her about her self-worth, she does not end up hating herself; in fact she ends up with self-respect.

Connecting with a safe person before and after a difficult event helps you to feel less alone. It often gives you the strength to take healthy risks during times when you might otherwise eat.

People with food and weight issues tend to turn to unsafe people for support, then clam up and get shy around safe people. Overeating and undereating are honest attempts to comfort ourselves when we don't know how to get comfort from people. Breaking isolation is therefore crucial to recovery. If you don't have any safe people in your life, we recommend that you contact Overeaters Anonymous to find a local meeting and/or seek out a therapist who meets the description of a safe person. If you are already seeing an individual psychotherapist, it could be very helpful for you to also join a therapy group.

Many people fear that reaching out for help is a sign of weakness. Yet, reaching out takes a lot of courage. It is not easy to go to another person, especially when we are feeling vulnerable, ashamed, hurt or confused. But reaching out helps us get past these feelings in a healthy manner. Reaching out is a way to resolve problems, and people who solve their problems end up feeling strong and confident, as well as connected to and intimate with others. Under these conditions, people find they do not have a need to turn to food for comfort.

❧ *Journey One*

Date:_____

1. Who are some potentially safe people in your life?

_____

_____

_____

_____

_____

_____

2. List ways in which you have recently reached out to and/or isolated from them :

Reached Out	Isolated
Called Carla and talked about my fear of gaining weight	*Watched TV and ate all weekend*

3. List ways in which the adults in your family reached out or isolated themselves:

Person	Reached Out	Isolated
Mom	*Didn't ever*	*Spent all day in bed when she was upset*

4. Complete the following sentences:
    a. What keeps me from reaching out is. . .

    _____

    _____

    _____

    b. If someone called and told me they were afraid of bothering me, but they had a problem they needed to talk about, I would think (or feel):

    _____

    _____

    _____

5. What are the reasons you give yourself for not deserving support from others?

    _____

    _____

    _____

6. Why do you deserve support from others?

    _____

    _____

    _____

❧ *Journey Two*

*Date:*_____

1. Who are some potentially safe people in your life?

_____

_____

_____

_____

_____

_____

2. List ways in which you have recently reached out to and/or isolated from them:

Reached Out	Isolated
Called Carla and talked about my fear of gaining weight	*Watched TV and ate all weekend*

3. Look back at Journey One, Question #2. How different or similar is your experience of reaching out to safe people now?

_____

_____

_____

_____

4. When do you isolate? What do you do when you isolate? Why do you think you isolate?

_____

_____

_____

_____

_____

5. List some things you could do to break your isolation.

_____

_____

_____

_____

_____

6. Think about when you first made a decision that people were not safe to reach out to. Write about this memory.

_____

_____

_____

_____

_____

7. Name the people in your life whom you continue to reach out to despite the fact that they are critical or unsupportive (unsafe).

_____

_____

_____

_____

_____

❧ *Journey Three*

*Date:*_____

1. Who are the people you reach out to when you need support?

_____

_____

_____

_____

_____

2. How have you changed regarding how much you reach out? (See Journeys One and Two.)

_____

_____

_____

_____

_____

_____

_____

3. Who are some potentially safe people that you would like to reach out to now?

_____

_____

_____

_____

_____

_____

_____

4. What keeps you from reaching out to them?

_____

_____

_____

_____

_____

_____

_____

_____

5. List ways you could reach out to them.

_____

_____

_____

_____

_____

_____

_____

_____

6. Pick one way you are willing to reach out to a safe person today. What could stop you? Will it stop you? What would encourage you?

_____

_____

_____

_____

_____

_____

_____

_____

Journey Four

*Date:*_____

1. Write about one time when you broke your isolation by reaching out to a safe person. What was it like? Prior to reaching out, what were you afraid of? Did your fears come true?

_____

_____

_____

_____

_____

_____

_____

2. What are the signs that you are isolating yourself from others? (As opposed to spending time alone or just being in a quiet or introspective mood).

_____

_____

_____

_____

_____

_____

3. When you isolate, what would be helpful to remember about reaching out?

_____

_____

_____

_____

_____

_____

4. Who are the safe people you have in your life today?

_____

_____

_____

_____

5.   a. Which people in your life are not safe?

_____

_____

_____

   b. Do you continue to reach out to them? Why?

_____

_____

_____

   c. What would it take for you to stop reaching out to them? What feelings do you think you would need to address?

_____

_____

_____

_____

_____

6. Look at Journey One, Question #1. How has your list of safe people changed?

_____

_____

_____

_____

7. Describe the ways in which you have become a safe person.

_____

_____

_____

_____

Chapter 3

Thoughts vs. Feelings

The word "feelings" will be used frequently throughout this workbook. That's because, in recovering from food, weight and body issues, it's as important to understand the use of this word as it is to understand the meaning of traffic lights. Like traffic lights, feelings tell us when to stop, when to yield, and when to go. Our feelings give us directions and warnings. If we don't heed our feelings, we miss out on vital information. Ignoring our feelings is like driving without paying attention to traffic lights and signs. Many of us live this way, without accessing our feelings. How do we do it? We rely on our thoughts. Although we may be very intelligent, with highly developed mental skills, when our minds are cut off from our feelings, our thoughts can become a liability.

Without crucial information from your feelings, your thoughts can mislead you. For example, you may feel physically hungry but not eat because you think you are fat or think you have to wait until noon. So you end up depriving yourself of nutrition when you actually need it. Or you may feel angry when someone mistreats you but not tell anyone because you think you're making too much of it, or because you think you'll only make them mad. In these cases, though the intent is to make yourself feel better, by relying on your thoughts and ignoring your feelings, you never solve the problems, and you end up feeling worse.

Thoughts are based on rules, beliefs, and judgments that we learn from others or personally invent. They are not necessarily based on fact. Feelings occur naturally and are experienced physically. While there are vast differences in people's thoughts and belief systems, everybody, everywhere, experiences the same primary feelings: happiness, sadness, anger, fear, loneliness, and hurt. Sometimes feelings are created by incorrect thinking. But they are still your feelings and need to be acknowledged and attended to.

Below are some common feelings to refer to as you continue your Journey. (We wouldn't want you driving a car without any headlights!) Each feeling is followed by variations within the same category. Notice there are two categories: Emotional feelings and Physical feelings.

Feelings Menu

Emotional:
1. Happy (peaceful, joyous, excited)
2. Sad (grieving, disappointed)
3. Angry (mad, frustrated, annoyed)
4. Ashamed (embarrassed, uncomfortable)
5. Proud (strong, righteous)
6. Afraid (nervous, anxious, terrified)
7. Loved (appreciated, cherished)
8. Loving (compassionate, accepting)
9. Hurt (wronged, victimized)
10. Lonely (empty, isolated)
11. Bored (indifferent, apathetic)

Physical:
1. Tired (sleepy, exhausted)
2. Energetic (hyper, restless)
3. Sick (achy, feverish)
4. Full (satisfied, stuffed)
5. Hungry (craving, starving)
6. Pained (sore, injured)
7. Sexual (sensual, longing)

How do you tell the difference between thoughts and feelings? Your feelings manifest in your body as physiological experiences and reactions. For example, when you are afraid, your stomach area may tighten, your heart rate may increase, or your whole body may stiffen. These physical experiences tell you that you are afraid. Likewise, when you're angry, your face may get flushed, and you may clench your jaw and/or your fists.

"Good" and "bad" are not feelings. They are judgments about feelings. They are what we think about our feelings. Let's say I'm feeling sad because I lost something. Suppose someone asks me how I'm doing and I say, "Bad." What I'm saying, then, both to the other person as well as to myself, is that I think my sad feeling is bad and that I shouldn't feel that way. But sadness is neither good nor bad. Sadness is a normal response to loss. It is as natural to feel sad at times as it is to feel happy. There are no good or bad feelings. Feelings just are. And did you know you could feel happy and sad at the same time? You can feel any number of, and any combination of, feelings all at once. You can even feel angry and loving in the same moment.

"Fat" is not a feeling. When we say "I feel fat," we are usually expressing a judgment. Sometimes we are referring to the body sensation of being "full," like after eating. But "full" is not the same as "fat." Other times, we are misinterpreting our emotions. We feel ashamed or we feel angry or anxious or upset and think it must be because we are "fat." We use the line "I feel fat" so readily that we forget to take the time to distinguish what we are really feeling.

Thinking we are "fat" can be a distraction we use to avoid — in much the same way as overeating or undereating — our feelings. Many of our clients begin their recovery thinking that "fat" is the only feeling they have. What a surprise when we inform them that "fat" is not a feeling at all!

The following is Marsea's story of how she learned to distinguish her feelings:

> *Early in my recovery I joined a therapy group. To begin each session, we each had to name three feelings we were experiencing at that moment. During my first few sessions I had no idea what I felt. It took hearing the other group members' feelings and comparing them to my own before I could figure out what mine were — hopefully by the time it was my turn! The counselor gave me a list of about 100 feelings and suggested that I study them. I carried the list and a notebook around with me and recorded my feelings throughout the day. I called it my crash course in Elementary Emotions 101. Writing down the words to describe my feelings helped me become aware of my inner self. Prior to that time, all I ever felt was "fine" or "fat" or "hungry." Without a language to express my feelings and my needs, I didn't know how to satisfy myself other than by eating, which, of course, never worked. Once I could name my feelings, I could write about them, talk about them and get help when I needed it. It was like learning the language in a foreign country — once you can speak some words, you can navigate and get what you need much more easily. Learning the language of feelings helped me to finally understand that a part of me was eating to stuff my feelings, while the rest of me was desperately in need of expressing them.*

It may be difficult for you to notice or recognize your feelings if you are accustomed to turning to food or obsessing about your weight every time your body begins to have an uncomfortable reaction. When we stuff our feelings down with food, drugs or alcohol, or hide them behind busyness, television, dieting, or other compulsive behaviors, we end up feeling numb. Numbness is not the absence of feelings, it is the absence of our connection to our feelings. Unfortunately, when we numb ourselves from certain feelings, we inadvertently numb ourselves from *all* of them. We don't get to pick and choose! Numbing often leads to depression. Depression means "pressing down" our feelings. When we are numb, our feelings are not available and we have to rely solely on our thoughts.

Thoughts are opinions. They are usually described in whole sentences, rather than one word, like feelings. For example, a thought sounds like this:

"I think he is absolutely wrong!" Or, "I shouldn't have acted like that."

We have a much better chance of resolving conflicts if we can identify the underlying feelings that are causing us to react. "I think he is absolutely wrong!" may be related to feelings of anger, and it might be more appropriate to go directly to the person and say what angered us and what we would prefer that person do. "I shouldn't have acted like that" may be connected to a feeling of shame. In that case, it would be more compassionate to say to yourself, "Boy, do I feel ashamed I did 'such and such.' What can I do to feel better about myself?" When we know what we're feeling we can communicate more directly and honestly. We also increase our chances of getting our needs met.

We have found that living life based solely on thinking prevents us from knowing what our bodies and souls really need in any given moment. When we don't know what we need, we often turn to food, or obsess about our weight. Dieting, or seeking out specific foods, become seemingly concrete solutions for problems that often don't have concrete or immediate answers. For example, if your thoughts are telling you you're doing poorly at your job, you might eat something in an attempt to soothe yourself. Perhaps what you really need is to talk to a friend, or co-worker, or boss, about your specific concerns. If your thoughts (judgments) prevent you from doing this, the problem remains unsolved.

Having unsettling feelings doesn't necessarily mean you need to do something. You may just need to sit with the anxiety until you can figure out a way to resolve the problem. Or maybe you need to let yourself feel anxious. An important part of recovering from food and weight issues is being willing to feel uncomfortable at times, rather than displacing the discomfort with food. When you use food to avoid troubling feelings, you end up with the original problem plus the additional problems of becoming physically uncomfortable from overeating, gaining weight, and feeling shame about yourself and your eating.

We have put a lot of emphasis on feelings in this chapter because most people with food and weight issues are inexperienced in this area. However, our ability to think things through is also very important. This is where our values and morals come in. There are times when we need to use our thinking to override our feelings in order for us to do what is right, but not necessarily what we feel like doing. For example, you find yourself attracted to someone. This does not mean you need to follow your feelings and jump into bed with that person. This is an instance where you need to take time to think about who this person is, how long you have known each other, whether or not you have the same goals and what the consequences could be of having a relationship. You also need to consider if having a sexual relationship fits into your own standards and goals.

Another example is when you are really angry or upset. This is usually not the best time to follow your feelings. We often need time to sit with strong emotions such as these and think about how we are going to react. It can be helpful to utilize our support system to help us think these things through.

Many people begin this Journey numb to their emotions, completely relying on their thoughts. Then, when they discover their feelings, they swing to the other extreme and think they need to honor every single feeling they have. True emotional health entails listening to both your head and your heart (your thoughts and your feelings). As you continue on your Journeys, practice noticing the difference between your thoughts and your feelings.

❧ *Journey One*

Date:_____

1. Write down the physiological (body) responses you have to each of these basic feelings:

1. Happy — *e.g. smiling, high energy*

_____

2. Sad

_____

3. Angry

_____

4. Ashamed

_____

5. Proud

_____

6. Afraid

_____

7. Loved

_____

8. Loving

_____

9. Hurt

_____

10. Lonely

_____

11. Bored

_____

2. Referring to the same list of feelings, write down your thoughts or judgments about each feeling.

    1. Happy

    e.g. "I should always be happy. Happy is a good feeling."

_____

    2. Sad

_____

    3. Angry

_____

    4. Ashamed

_____

    5. Proud

_____

    6. Afraid

_____

    7. Loved

_____

    8. Loving

_____

    9. Hurt

_____

    10. Lonely

_____

    11. Bored

_____

3. Go back to the above list and write down the names of the people who taught you those beliefs and judgments.

4. List below as many feelings as you can identify in yourself right now. (Most feelings are one word.) Take time to pay attention to your body and to allow the feelings to become clear. Remember, there are no good or bad feelings, and "fat" is not a feeling!

_____

_____

_____

_____

_____

_____

5. What is it like for you to focus on and identify your feelings?

_____

_____

_____

_____

_____

_____

_____

6. How many times a day do you think you "feel fat"?

_____

This sign designates what we will call a *Spontaneous Road Trip*. A Spontaneous Road Trip is akin to deciding to go off the beaten path and explore unknown territory. When you arrive at this sign in your workbook, we encourage you to do whatever you want on this page. You can use it to express anything that's going on for you at this time. You can draw, write spontaneously about your thoughts and feelings, make a collage, write a poem, insert a photograph of yourself... anything that will help you explore and record this current part of your Journey. (Remember, there is no right or wrong way to do this!)

❧ *Journey Two*

*Date:*_____

1. List below as many feelings as you can identify in yourself right now. (Note where in your body you feel each one.)

_____

_____

_____

_____

_____

_____

2. Which feelings are you judging and which are you accepting?

_____

_____

_____

_____

_____

_____

3. List times this week when you listened to your feelings, and times when you ignored them.

_____

_____

_____

_____

_____

_____

_____

4. Describe the consequences of judging your feelings vs. accepting them. What happens in each case?

_____

_____

_____

_____

_____

_____

_____

5. Think about the last time you used "fat" to describe your feelings. What do you think you were actually feeling at the time?

_____

_____

_____

_____

_____

_____

_____

6. How many times a day do you use the word "fat" to describe your feelings? Go back to Journey One, Question #6 and review what you wrote back then.

_____

❧ *Journey Three*

*Date:*_____

1. List below as many feelings as you can identify in yourself right now. (Distinguish which ones are physical and which ones are emotional.)

> e.g.   *Tired (physical)*
> *Sad (emotional)*

_____

_____

_____

_____

_____

_____

2. What is it like to identify your feelings now compared to Journey One?

_____

_____

_____

_____

_____

_____

3. What thoughts might be getting in the way of dealing with your feelings?

_____

_____

_____

_____

4. Identify as many times as you can recall during the past 24 hours when you communicated your feelings to another person.

_____

_____

_____

_____

_____

_____

5. Which of the above feelings would you have previously eaten over?

_____

_____

_____

_____

_____

_____

6. How often do you use the word "fat" to describe your feelings? Reread Journeys One and Two, Question #6, and write about how you have or haven't changed.

_____

_____

_____

_____

_____

_____

❦ *Journey Four*

Date:_____

1. What have you learned about your emotions that you didn't know before you began your work in this book?

_____

_____

_____

_____

_____

_____

2. List below all the feelings which you are experiencing right now.

_____

_____

_____

_____

_____

_____

3. Write in as much detail as you can about each of the feelings you listed above. (Use extra paper if necessary).

_____

_____

_____

_____

_____

_____

_____

4. What was it like for you to write about your feelings?

_____

_____

_____

_____

_____

_____

5. What thoughts or judgments are you aware of regarding your feelings? List the thoughts that prevent you from truly feeling your feelings.

_____

_____

_____

_____

_____

_____

_____

6. Pick a feeling that is difficult for you to allow yourself to feel and write what a very loving person would say to you about that feeling.

Feeling: _____

Loving Response: _____

_____

_____

_____

_____

_____

_____

Chapter 4

Stuffing vs. Acknowledging Feelings

Normally, feelings flow through us like clouds drifting by in the sky. Sadness, joy, fear and peace come and go in varying degrees at different speeds throughout our days. When we're on a road trip we have to deal with and adjust our plans according to the weather. While we would never think we could actually control the weather, we most certainly try to control our feelings. Those of us with food and weight issues don't let our feelings drift by like clouds, simply noticing them, or perhaps commenting on their form and dimension. Instead, we try to construct walls to hold them back, or we bury them deep inside, or we strive to change them into something they're not. Often we critically judge ourselves with thoughts like, "I'm such a crybaby" or "I'm really losing it."

Abusing food and obsessing on our bodies are some of the many ways we attempt to achieve these unacknowledged goals of controlling our feelings. Most of our parents used food to cheer us up. It works, doesn't it? But at what cost? Every time a cookie is used to transform anger into a smile, the message to the anger is: "Go away! You are bad! You shouldn't exist! I can't handle you!" Where, then, does the anger go? One of two places: a) It gets stored inside your body, or b) It gets vented at the wrong people, including yourself!

If you try to stuff your anger it does not just go away. Anger is an important feeling. It tells us when something isn't right, when we or others are being violated, or when we have been hurt or scared. It's important that we listen to our anger. The same is true for other feelings, as well. Sadness, fear, and happiness all have reasons for surfacing when they do, and it is critical that we listen to their messages.

Food does not get rid of feelings. When we try to use food in this way, there is never enough of it to do the job. Those of us who have problems with food often do not know what we feel or how food and feelings could possibly be connected. Usually, the connection isn't made until we begin to admit that food and weight are not our only problems. It's only then that we begin to discover the multitude and intensity of feelings that we have when we don't use food to numb, blunt or stuff them back down.

Andrea:

Before recovery, I didn't know I was "stuffing" feelings. I thought I just needed to eat. I thought eating just the right food, or combinations of food, would make me feel better, would fill my insatiable emptiness. Now that I understand the truth about my eating disorder, I can see with compassion that every time I overate, I was having feelings that I didn't know what to do with. I didn't know it was okay to be sad and to cry. I didn't know it was okay to be anxious and to talk about it and get support. Eating excess food was an attempt to help me avoid my uncomfortable feelings. I was "fine" to people on the outside, while inside I was hating myself for overeating and still troubled by the unacknowledged feelings.

Today I know the incredible power of acknowledging my feelings. Sometimes that means telling my truth to the person I am with, sometimes it means telling it to a safe person, and sometimes it means just acknowledging it to myself. When I share my feelings with other people, I often find out that what I think they are thinking is not at all what they are thinking. In other words: I'm not the world's best mind-reader! You would not believe all the excess food I consumed over things I thought people were thinking about me. (Well, maybe you would!)

When my husband, Michael, and I were first dating, we went to a concert out of town. We didn't have time to stop for dinner before the show so I had offered to pack us a meal to eat on the way. He suggested that he drive first while I ate and then we'd switch seats so he could eat while I finished the drive. I went with the plan and began eating my dinner in the passenger seat. He kept looking over at me and my food, and I began to feel very insecure and ashamed. I also began to do a lot of mind-reading, none of it complimentary. I have no doubt that the old me would have stuffed down those feelings, telling myself, "It's easy — don't say a word, eat faster, have butterflies in your stomach and a face red with shame. Then be quiet and distant the whole night and binge and purge as soon as you get home."

Well, the new me decided to take a risk and tell him what I was thinking and feeling. "I think you're thinking all these negative things about me right now and I am full of shame and want to puke" was about the best I could come up with at the time. "What do you think I'm thinking?" he lovingly asked. "That I'm eating too much and too fast and that I'm too fat to be eating all this food. And that I'm taking too big bites." Michael said, "Oh, honey, I'm just looking over to see how long until you'll be finished because the food looks great and I can't wait for it to be my turn." Now, I never would have come up with that! If I hadn't honored my feelings and spoken up, I wouldn't have received the incredible relief I experienced that evening in the car, not to mention the closeness it created between me and Michael as we laughed over the whole thing.

Learning how to acknowledge uncomfortable feelings is one of the most important skills you need on your Journey of Recovery. Acknowledging your feelings does not necessarily mean that you have to do something about them. It does mean that you notice them. Just like signs on the road, it's important that you see them even if you don't attend to every one. A sign that advertises a restaurant ahead may only be important if you are hungry and you like that restaurant. A sign that says STOP, however, must be obeyed immediately or there could be disastrous consequences.

Joan, a client of ours, was at work one day when a co-worker made a derogatory comment about Joan's work. Joan felt very angry, but didn't think it would be appropriate to say something at the time. By acknowledging to herself how inappropriate the co-worker's statement was and promising herself to express her feelings about it to her friends when she got home, and possibly her co-worker later, she was able to make it through the day without using food to stuff down her anger. She repeated to herself throughout the day, "You have a right to be angry, that was an inappropriate, insulting remark."

Carol, on the other hand, had an experience where she acknowledged her feelings and chose to say something about it on the spot. She was on a first date and the man she was with put his arm around her. She was very uncomfortable. In the past she would not have said anything. This time, however, she spoke up and told the man it was too soon for physical touch. It was an awkward moment, but he did remove his arm. Carol responded to her feelings and also had the opportunity to see how her date responded to her feelings. If he hadn't been respectful, that would have been very important information for her to discover.

Once you acknowledge your feelings (which doesn't necessarily mean that you like them), you are then in a position to decide whether or not to take action. Sometimes it's important to do or say something, while at other times it's just as important to not say anything. Privacy is healthy; it is okay to choose not to share certain things with certain people. It's secrecy you want to watch out for. Those of us with food, weight, and body image issues tend to keep secrets due to embarrassment or shame. Keeping secrets then perpetuates the feeling of shame. It's a vicious cycle. If we never talk about the things of which we are ashamed, we never get the opportunity to receive compassion, understanding, or the help we may desperately need.

Of course, it's okay to be private about certain things. We are not advocating that you go around telling everybody everything. Your feelings are precious and need to be shared with safe, supportive people who will hear them and not judge or criticize you. Privacy means having healthy boundaries about who and what and how much to tell. It's a decision that comes from maturity and self-respect.

Secrets tend to be unhealthy, coming from a belief that we are "bad" and unforgivable. Secrets contribute to our need to overeat or undereat, which can then create more secrets. Many of our clients tell us that their spouses, partners, and closest friends had no idea they suffered from a serious eating disorder. The secrecy aided them in their self-destruction.

As we begin to decrease our secret behaviors with food, many of us discover that we have feelings that we have kept secret for a very long time. And some of us find we even begin to remember events from our past that had felt so shameful we had "forgotten" about them. As we begin to reveal and heal our secret histories and feelings, our secret behaviors with food diminish.

A good indicator that you may be keeping a secret (as opposed to a private thought or feeling) is if it is laced with a feeling of shame and a belief that you cannot tell anybody. When something is private, you have a choice about telling people. You are not bound by shame. An example of distinguishing between secrecy and privacy is illustrated by Brenda, one of our clients. Brenda revealed in therapy that when she was nine years old her uncle had repeatedly fondled her breasts. He told her not to tell anyone, and, believing it was partially her fault, she never did. For thirty years she kept the secret, was ashamed of her body, distrustful of men, and driven to eat excess food.

Having finally shared her secret in therapy, Brenda was able to get the support and understanding she needed in order to heal her shame. She eventually found that she felt comfortable sharing this unpleasant part of her past with a few of her friends. There were other people in her life, however, whom she chose not to tell. This was a healthy decision to maintain her privacy.

Revealing a secret to the right person can be extremely healing. You often find out that you are not alone, that other people feel or have felt as you do. Remember the "Same Brain Theory" — the same brain that has food, weight, and body image issues needs help from other, healthier, brains in order to change its patterns. We often need the perspective, compassion, or forgiveness of other people in order to move through painful emotions.

Although many people openly share certain thoughts about their food and weight, such as, "I feel so fat," or "I ate like a pig," or "I just started a new diet," rarely do the same people express (or even know) what is really going on internally. Often, these statements are masking mental anguish and deep pain. Rarely do we tell a friend the truth, such as, "I feel so afraid and out of control" or "I feel so confused and depressed." Sadly, it is more socially acceptable to say, "I'm so fat! I've got to get back on my diet."

For now, we ask you to focus on just noticing your feelings; they are the lifesaving signs on your Journey. Notice when you are stuffing them and when you are acknowledging them. Notice when you are being real with people and when you are not being authentic.

❧ *Journey One*

*Date:*_____

1. Think through your day today, starting with when you woke up. List every feeling you can remember having. (Most feelings are one word, such as happy, sad, scared, mad. And don't forget, "fat" is not a feeling!)

_____

_____

_____

_____

_____

2. Without being judgmental, what do you notice about your list?

_____

_____

_____

_____

_____

_____

3. Pick three feelings from your list and draw them here as clouds. (No artistic skills necessary. If you feel anxious about the outcome, use your opposite hand; this removes the pressure.)

4. What secrets are you keeping right now? (You can use shorthand or vague notes as a way of maintaining your privacy, if necessary.)

_____

_____

_____

_____

_____

_____

5. Put a letter "P" by the things on your above list that seem appropriate to keep private, and an "S" by those you keep secret due to shame or fear.

6. List the various ways in which you hide or stuff your feelings. (i.e. smiling when mad, overtalking, getting silent, excessive TV watching...)

_____

_____

_____

_____

_____

_____

7. Describe how you stuffed or acknowledged your feelings today? Which feelings were these?

_____

_____

_____

_____

_____

_____

_____

❦ *Journey Two*

Date: _____

1. Think through your day today, starting with when you woke up. List every feeling you can remember having. (Most feelings are one word, such as happy, sad, scared or mad. Remember "fat" is not a feeling!)

_____

_____

_____

_____

_____

_____

2. Without being judgmental, what do you notice about your list?

_____

_____

_____

_____

_____

_____

3. How did/do feelings get stuffed or acknowledged in your family?

_____

_____

_____

_____

_____

_____

4. In what ways did you either stuff or acknowledge your feelings today?

_____

_____

_____

_____

_____

_____

_____

5. Pick a feeling that you frequently eat over. Imagine that a little girl you cared about came to you and told you she felt that same feeling right now. How would you treat her?

_____

_____

_____

_____

_____

_____

_____

6. Look at Question #4 in Journey One. Have you told anyone any of the things on your list? If not, why not? If you did, how did it go?

_____

_____

_____

_____

_____

_____

_____

Journey Three

*Date:*_____

1. Think through your day today, starting with when you woke up. List every feeling you can remember having. (Remember, most feelings are one word! e.g. happy, sad, scared, mad.)

_____

_____

_____

_____

_____

_____

_____

2. Without being judgmental, what do you notice about your list?

_____

_____

_____

_____

_____

_____

_____

3. In what ways did you either stuff or acknowledge your feelings today?

_____

_____

_____

_____

_____

_____

_____

4. Reflecting back on Journey One and Journey Two, how do you deal with your feelings now compared to how you dealt with them then?

_____

_____

_____

_____

_____

_____

_____

5. Make a list of any secrets you are currently keeping.

_____

_____

_____

_____

_____

_____

6.   a. Who would be potentially safe to tell any of these secrets to?

_____

    b. How would you like them to respond, if you told them?

_____

_____

    c. How are you affected by keeping these secrets?

_____

_____

    d. What do you think will happen if you keep these secrets?

_____

_____

_____

This sign designates what we will call a Spontaneous Road Trip. A Spontaneous Road Trip is akin to deciding to go off the beaten path and explore unknown territory. When you arrive at this sign in your workbook, we encourage you to do whatever you want on this page. You can use it to express anything that's going on for you at this time. You can draw, write spontaneously about your thoughts and feelings, make a collage, write a poem, insert a photograph of yourself... anything that will help you explore and record this current part of your Journey. (Remember there is no right or wrong way to do this!)

❧ *Journey Four*

Date:_____

1. List below any feelings you have been stuffing.

_____

_____

_____

_____

2. What do you guess are the reasons you have been stuffing each of the above feelings?

_____

_____

_____

_____

_____

_____

_____

3. How could you make yourself feel comfortable and safe enough to express them?

_____

_____

_____

_____

_____

_____

4. List some of the methods you use to stuff your feelings.

_____

_____

_____

_____

5. Look back at Journey Three, Questions #5 and #6. What has happened with the secrets you wrote about?

_____

_____

_____

_____

_____

_____

6. List some occasions when you think it's appropriate to withhold your feelings.

_____

_____

_____

_____

_____

_____

7. Write about some of the benefits you have received from expressing your difficult feelings to safe people.

_____

_____

_____

_____

_____

_____

_____

_____

_____

_____

Chapter 5

Aggressive vs. Assertive Communication

Now that you're learning to acknowledge your feelings, you'll find that there are times when you need to communicate them to other people. This chapter will teach you the difference between communicating aggressively and communicating assertively.

If you have been abusing food or your body for many years, you have that many years of unexpressed feelings within you. You may feel like a volcano, ready to explode. Once you stop stuffing your feelings down with food, you might be inclined to express them aggressively, especially if that is what you witnessed in your family. Or you may be so afraid of hurting someone with your feelings that you are tempted to revert back to stuffing them down with food. Like most of us, you probably had no model for communicating your feelings in an assertive way. If the people in your family had lovingly and assertively communicated their feelings, and encouraged you to do the same, you probably wouldn't have had to stuff your feelings in the first place.

So here you are now, committed to learning a new way to communicate, a way that lies somewhere between stuffing your feelings altogether and erupting like a volcano. What other options do you have? You can communicate your feelings through *Indirect Communication* (writing or speaking to an uninvolved safe person), or *Direct Communication* (speaking directly to the person who is involved). Or, you may want to use both.

Like many, you may choose Indirect Communication first, for the following reasons:
- Fear — of rejection, of an unknown outcome, of conflict, or of hurting someone.
- Not knowing what to say, or how to word it lovingly.
- Feeling too angry to communicate respectfully.
- The person with whom you need to communicate may be unsafe or unavailable.
- The person you have conflict with is deceased.

These are all valid reasons for taking the indirect route.

One way to express feelings indirectly is to write them out. Writing can help you release feelings you have been holding in. Remember, you can either stuff your feelings down with food, or you can let them out. Writing is one way to let them out safely. Often, writing releases much of the emotion and frees you up to approach the person directly, in a calmer way than before. You can write in a journal, notebook, or on loose paper. You can also write a series of letters to the person with whom you have a problem (letters which you will **not** be sending). In these letters, give yourself the opportunity to express all your feelings, without restraint. We recommend that you try not to judge or censor yourself in these letters — write down anything that comes to mind. Write as many letters as you need until you've said everything that you feel. (Remember, it is important to respect and protect both your feelings and the other person's by disposing of the letters or making sure they are safely stored.) Sometimes one letter will be enough, other times you will need to write many. You can write a letter every day, if you want. Write until you have achieved clarity, serenity, or at least some relief.

Another way to express feelings indirectly is to talk to someone who is safe and objective (see "safe people," pg. 29). Let's say you realize you feel hurt about something a friend has said. You decide you are not going to eat over this, but you don't know what else to do. So you first talk to someone else, a safe and objective person. (In order to avoid gossiping, you can refrain from using any names or identifying descriptions.) After expressing to this person all the feelings that were bothering you, you may find that you feel better and there is no need to further express your feelings.

Then again, you may discover there are things you need to say directly in order for you to feel complete and be assured that the person understands what was hurtful to you. This can be scary and challenging, but if you want intimate relationships with people, rather than with food, being assertive is part of the Journey. Of course, how you express your feelings is very important.

A person communicating aggressively: yells, blames, attacks, criticizes. The goal in Aggressive Communication is to win, even if it's at the expense of others. And while the person who communicates aggressively may momentarily feel better after discharging her feelings, the people on the receiving end usually feel worse. Aggressive Communication destroys relationships and is, therefore, a dead-end road.

Assertive Communication, on the other hand, can heal and deepen relationships. It is an open-ended road that can lead to greater intimacy. A person who communicates assertively is: honest, direct, respectful, open-minded. The assertive communicator's goal is to resolve a problem so that both people win. Because it honors the other person's feelings, assertive communication creates opportunities for negotiation and intimacy. Although there may be some initial awkwardness and discomfort, once conflicts are resolved, the people involved usually feel much closer.

When you need to approach someone directly, one set of skills that can help you assertively address problems is *Loving Confrontation*. Loving Confrontation is a way to approach a problem with another person in a direct, healthy, responsible manner. The intention of a Loving Confrontation is to heal the relationship problem, rather than to aggressively vent feelings. (You can vent feelings indirectly by writing or talking with your uninvolved safe person.) Loving Confrontation is a way to be respectful and productive in solving a problem with another person. You don't have to feel loving toward the person. Loving Confrontation is about loving yourself enough to handle your problems and to do so with integrity. When you handle your problems with integrity, you gain respect for yourself. Following are four steps to a successful Loving Confrontation.

Step One: Make a Plan

If you are new to Assertive Communication, you may not be able to remember how to do it in the heat of the moment. It's okay to tell someone you need some time to think through your feelings before discussing the situation. Assertive Communication does not necessarily come naturally; therefore it is useful to take the time to plan out what you are going to say. Your goal is to communicate lovingly and assertively. If you are particularly angry or hurt, you may need time to calm down. You may also need help from a supportive person in order to find a loving way to articulate what is bothering you. It can help to write your feelings down, and then decide what you want to say and how you want to say it.

Planning helps you separate your current problems from your unresolved family or childhood issues. Let's say an incident with your friend was emotionally charged. After reflecting on it for awhile you realize your reaction was so strong because the situation reminded you of a similar pattern with your mother. If you had just picked up the phone and called your friend without thinking about it, your automatic response might have been the same as if she were your mom. You might have found yourself reacting angrily with aggression, or perhaps in a childlike or passive manner. By taking the time to sort through your feelings and making a plan for communicating them, you may be able to discover that only part of the issue really had to do with your friend. In order to avoid automatic responses, it helps to work through the emotionally charged issues via Indirect Communication methods, such as writing or talking to safe people in your support system.

Another part of making a plan is scheduling the time to talk. It is important to be respectful of the other person's time and feelings. You wouldn't want to call someone right before work, begin a discussion on a difficult issue, and leave the person to struggle emotionally all day. Finding a mutual good time is part of being loving. It also gives the other person a chance to prepare or get support.

Step Two: Tell Your Truth

Telling your truth means speaking from your heart, saying what feels true for you in the moment. It is important that you do this in a kind, unhurtful, manner. Sometimes, in the beginning, it's really hard to know how to do this, especially if for years you haven't been paying attention to your own truth. You may have been stuffing your truth down with food, starving it through dieting, and deflecting it with body hatred.

In the Transition and Early Recovery stages it can help to have some guidelines. One method we suggest is known as "Direct I Statements." With this structure, you complete the following four sentences:

- I see . . .   (What you have observed or noticed. Be as objective and brief as possible.)
- I think . . .   (What your interpretation is.)

• I feel . . .   (Use one-word feelings. See page 41 if you need some help.)
• I need . . .   (What you would like the person to do instead.)

Here's an example of using Direct I Statements:
"Mary, I see that you have been late the past several times we've gotten together. I think it means that our dates aren't important to you, and that leaves me feeling hurt. I need to know that I matter to you, so I need you to make sure you arrive on time or else call me when you're running late."

Another structure is: "When you/I feel . . ." Here you fill in these three sentences:

• When you . . .
• I feel . . .
• And I would prefer . . .

This would sound like:
"Mary, when you come late to our meetings, I feel hurt and angry, and I would prefer that you arrive on time or call me if you're running late."

In telling your truth, it works best to be as brief and to the point as possible. Otherwise, your message may be unclear or may get lost in your words.

In Ongoing Recovery, you probably won't need to rely on such specific structures. Your challenge in this stage is to just be lovingly honest and speak from your heart.

Step Three: Listen to the Response

Sometimes this step seems like the hardest one because being direct about our feelings can create a reaction in the other person. Of course, there are times when the other person is glad you said something and the exchange draws you closer. But people can also respond with hurt, anger, or defensiveness.

Remember, what you want is a Loving Confrontation. So it's really important to stay centered. It helps to focus on your breathing as a way to relax and to concentrate on understanding what the other person is feeling. This is very different than aggressively trying to get your point across. Once you have said what you planned to say, the best thing to do is to be quiet and listen.

If the other person is disrespectful in his or her response, return to the format and address what is happening now. For example: "When you yell at me like this, I feel scared and upset, and I would prefer it if you would find a way to discuss this with me rather than yell at me." If he or she remains aggressive or becomes abusive, then you can say something like, "I'm not willing to continue until you can be polite, or loving or rational. . ." Then leave.

But assuming your friend/relative/acquaintance is not abusive and you're going to talk the issue through, it is important to give him/her the respect that you would want. Respect means really listening. You want to make sure the other person feels heard. You can do this by asking questions. Try not to argue. Let them express their feelings in the same way you want them to allow you to express yours. The more comfortable you get in allowing yourself to feel and express your feelings, the more comfortable you will become in allowing others to have their feelings. With practice, this will get easier!

As you listen, try to understand others' feelings, their concerns, and their points of view. This will help you in the fourth, and final step, which follows.

Step Four: Work on Solutions

Often in relationships we have problems with something a friend or a relative is doing and we don't say a word. Instead we turn to food and stay resentful or hurt. But Loving Confrontations, and all the Journeys in this book, are about healing and having genuine relationships with people, rather than food. Many times we can restore relationships through negotiating and finding common ground.

The last step in this process is to offer a solution and be open to a counterproposal. For instance, to the friend who chronically keeps you waiting, you might suggest, "How about if you call me if you're going to be late so that I don't rush to our dates."

Your friend might answer, "OK, that sounds good," or "Actually, I want to make a commitment not to be late anymore," or "I can call you on Tuesdays but on Thursdays I'm not near a phone." With proposals and counterproposals you can keep negotiations flexible. You might say, "Let's try this for a month, then reevaluate."

The above four steps to a Loving Confrontation (Make a Plan, Tell Your Truth, Listen to the Response, and Work on Solutions) are meant to be guidelines. There is no one right way. In the beginning, Loving Confrontations may be awkward, but they become natural over time. Because you are dealing with people, there will always be variations based on personalities, situations, and where each of you are in your own growth process.

Here's an example of how Andrea and Marsea handled a Loving Confrontation:

Andrea:

> *Over ten years ago when Marsea and I first became friends, we were both beginning our Journeys of recovery from food and weight issues. I had been telling Marsea a lot about myself, but I felt insecure because she was not sharing equally of herself. Although I liked that Marsea was a good friend and listener, I worried that I was talking too much. I felt vulnerable after our visits, having told her many personal things while she had not revealed much about herself. I started to think she was judging me. I decided to bring up my discomfort in a Loving Confrontation.*
>
> *I made a plan. (In this case I chose not to talk to anybody or write it through.) The issue seemed simple enough that I believed I could approach Marsea directly. We had arranged to go to a movie, and I planned to bring up my feelings afterward when we were in the car together.*
>
> *When the time arrived, I told her I needed to speak to her about something and asked if she was open to it. I also told her I felt really scared. When she said "yes" I used the When You/I Feel Format. To the best of my*

recollection it went something like this: "When you and I are together, the amount of sharing I do compared to what you do doesn't seem even. I feel ashamed and insecure about it. I would prefer it if you would share more about yourself when we're together and tell me what you're thinking after I've shared something personal."

Marsea:

When Andrea brought up the topic, I felt embarrassed and self-conscious. I knew she was right about the imbalance in our relationship, but I was scared to open up more. In her Loving Confrontation, Andrea hadn't judged me or criticized me and I was grateful for that. I knew by the tone of her voice that she cared about me and our friendship. Although I felt a little defensive, I made an effort to respond honestly.

Andrea:

Marsea indicated that she understood my feelings and she apologized for not being more open. Then she told me about her family. She said that when she was younger they never showed much interest in what she had to say. So, basically, Marsea decided at an early age that people didn't care about what she thought. I was really surprised and sad for her because I had great respect for Marsea's thoughts. I wished she had experienced more interest from her family.

I would never have learned so much about Marsea if I hadn't brought up the subject of sharing our thoughts and feelings with each other. Now I understood her so much better. My big fear that she would say, "Yes, you do talk too much," was alleviated. What a relief to know Marsea's silences were about her and her history, not about me.

I asked Marsea if she would like us to work together on this, and if so, I could encourage her to share more on a personal level by asking her questions.

Marsea:

I thought that was a good idea. The fact that Andrea wanted to know more about me, and was willing to help me open up, really touched me. However, I didn't want to burden her with the whole responsibility so I said I would work on pushing myself to share more as well. I also proposed that when I felt self-conscious or needed reassurance about whether she was really interested, I would check in with her by asking, "Do you really want to hear this?"

Andrea:

> *I'm really glad I asserted myself. Had I not, I probably would have begun to share less with Marsea and we would have become more distant, perhaps eventually drifting apart.*

Marsea:

> *And I'm grateful to Andrea for taking the risk of confronting me. If she hadn't brought up her feelings, I probably would have continued in my role as a listener, a role I took on in most of my relationships. As a result of her Loving Confrontation, I became more open and outspoken in all of my relationships. What seemed like a risky subject turned into a growth experience for both of us.*

❧ *Journey One*

*Date:*_____

1. How did each member of your immediate family express his/her feelings? Aggressively, assertively, or not at all?

_____

_____

_____

_____

_____

_____

2. List the people about whom you are currently stuffing your feelings.

_____

_____

_____

3. Pick one person from the above list and, on a separate piece of paper, write an aggressive letter to that person. You can say anything you want in this letter without regard to his/her feelings. (You won't send this. Make sure you keep the letter in a safe place or destroy it.)

4. Now write another letter to the same person. But this time use Step Two of the Loving Confrontation (pg. 69). In this letter we encourage you to tell your truth in a direct, loving, respectful manner.

5. After writing both letters, describe here how you are feeling right now.

_____

_____

_____

_____

_____

🌿 *Journey Two*

Date:_____

1. a. Describe the last time someone communicated aggressively with you.

    _____

    _____

    _____

    _____

    _____

    b. Describe the last time someone was assertive in his/her communication with you.

    _____

    _____

    _____

    _____

    _____

    c. What felt different? What effect, if any, did each experience have on your eating?

    _____

    _____

    _____

    _____

    _____

2. a. Describe the last time you were aggressive in your communication with someone.

    _____

    _____

    _____

    _____

    _____

b. Describe the last time you were assertive with someone.

_____

_____

_____

_____

_____

c. What felt different? What effect, if any, did each experience have on your eating?

_____

_____

_____

_____

_____

3. List the people about whom you are currently stuffing your feelings.

_____

_____

_____

4. Compare this list to Question #2, Journey One. Are you stuffing your feelings about more or fewer people?

_____

5. List your fears about being assertive.

_____

_____

_____

_____

❧ *Journey Three*

*Date:*_____

1. Make a list of all the people about whom you are currently stuffing your feelings.

_____

_____

_____

_____

_____

_____

2. On a separate piece of paper, write an aggressive letter to each person on your list.

3. On a separate piece of paper, write an assertive letter to each person, using Step Two of the Loving Confrontation format, which is to tell your truth. (See pg. 69 for help.)

4.   a. Which situations feel resolved after writing these letters? In which do you need to seek help, or go further with an actual Loving Confrontation?

_____

_____

_____

_____

_____

_____

b. What will it take for you to do a Loving Confrontation with one of these people?

_____

_____

_____

_____

_____

_____

5. a. What are your fears about doing Loving Confrontations?

_____

_____

_____

_____

_____

b. What are your fears about not doing Loving Confrontations?

_____

_____

_____

_____

_____

c. What price do you pay when you avoid confronting people?

_____

_____

_____

_____

_____

_____

❧ *Journey Four*

Date:_____

1. Who are your current role models for assertive communication?

_____

_____

_____

_____

2. Where on the scale do you see yourself when confronted by a difficult situation?

passive   *assertive*   *aggressive*
(withdrawn)

3. What would it take for you to move one notch closer to the center?

_____

_____

_____

_____

_____

4. Write about a recent situation in which you were either passive or aggressive.

_____

_____

_____

_____

_____

_____

_____

5. How would an assertive person have handled that situation? Write in detail what they would have said or done.

_____

_____

_____

_____

_____

_____

6. How do you feel after you have been either passive or aggressive?

_____

_____

_____

_____

_____

_____

7. How do you feel after you have been assertive?

_____

_____

_____

_____

_____

_____

8. What do you think you would need in order to act more assertively?

_____

_____

_____

_____

_____

Chapter 6

Criticism vs. Praise

Have you ever noticed how you speak to yourself? Day-in and day-out we are all having internal conversations with ourselves. The tone of these contributes greatly to how we end up feeling. Once we start paying attention to our inner conversations, we are often shocked at the amount of criticism we give ourselves. We learn that though we may be very kind and loving toward others, to ourselves we are cruel, unforgiving, and even abusive. Harsh words can sting as much as a slap in the face, and many of us spend entire days berating ourselves.

As we look back on our lives, many of us recall teachers admonishing us to do better, or telling us that we had "so much potential" when we thought we were doing our best. Coaches may have told us we weren't good enough for the team or that we needed to run faster, jump higher, lose weight or gain it. Our parents may have told us we should be nicer to our siblings, get higher grades, eat more or eat less. Peers may have teased us about our weight or our appearance. Did we ever get to hear that we were doing well? Or that we were fine exactly the way we were? If we were excited or bubbly, our parents may have told us to calm down. If we were quiet or shy, people may have tried to pull us "out of our shell." In each of these instances, the message to us was that we were not good enough the way we were; we needed to change or improve ourselves. There are certainly times when assessments or feedback are appropriate, but only if they're balanced with positive messages and an appreciation of who we are. Shaming statements are never helpful, they only make us feel ashamed.

When there is more criticism than praise, children tend to remember the criticism and forget the praise. Children desperately want, and need, approval. When they get criticized instead, it can be devastating. In many families, critical responsiveness may have been passed down from generation to generation. Many of our parents simply gave us what they had been given. They criticized us in an attempt to help us become better people, in the same way their parents criticized them to try to help them become better people. We now know that shaming children is harmful and counterproductive. Children who are well-behaved because they are fearful of criticism become adults who lack confidence and self-esteem.

Children who lack kindness and positive attention in their lives often turn to sugar as a way of nurturing themselves. This pattern gets carried into adulthood. Many of our clients come to realize that with constant self-criticism running through their minds, the only "sweetness" in their lives comes from the sugar they consume. It is essential that you find non sugar-related ways to experience sweetness in your life. Bubble baths, massages, manicures, juicy novels, sexual intimacy, and heart-to-heart talks are some ways to provide yourself with sweetness. There is nothing inherently wrong with eating sugar, but if you don't have sweetness in your day to day life, you become vulnerable to having an addictive and unfulfilling relationship with it.

There seems to be a common theme among many of our clients who feel that if they were to treat themselves sweetly, and praise rather than criticize themselves, they would become lazy, vain, or conceited. That's just not the case. We have found that when we treat ourselves kindly we feel better, have more energy, and have more satisfying relationships.

Self-criticism often results in an inability to accept praise from other people as well: "Oh, it was nothing," "What, this old rag?" "The turkey is not that good, I overcooked it." Self-criticism causes distance between us and others because we fail to accept their kind words or positive feelings about us.

What if we were to tell you that praise is nourishing? If you starve yourself of praise, your soul gets very hungry. Sometimes we try to fill that hunger with food when what we really need is appreciation for who we are and what we have done. Receiving praise, from yourself and others, is like giving your car a regular oil change; it is necessary to keep your gears running smoothly.

Marsea:

"I slept too late... I should get up earlier... I shouldn't have eaten so much last night... I'm so fat I have nothing to wear today... I shouldn't eat breakfast... I've got to lose weight... I look terrible... I should exercise for at least an hour today... I'm so lazy."

These are the thoughts I used to wake up to every morning. What a way to start the day! Miserable and depressed, the only praise I ever gave myself was for not eating. I believed that my self-criticism was useful — that it was helping me to maintain control. I failed to see that not only was it not working, it was contributing to my feelings of unhappiness and worthlessness.

One day, in my support group, I heard the phrase, "Stop 'shoulding' on yourself!" and I began to notice how many of my thoughts were based on 'shoulds.' I decided to experiment with dropping the word 'should' from my vocabulary. Every time I heard myself use it, I'd change it to the word 'could' and I noticed how different that felt. Instead of saying to myself, "It's warm out, I should be outside," I would say, "It's warm out and I could go outside, but I think I'd rather stay in right now."

Eventually I stopped "shoulding on myself." This change in my internal vocabulary had profound effects on me. I started feeling more gentle toward myself, softer. I didn't feel quite so tense and driven. I was able to relax more, and, ironically, I was getting more accomplished than before. I started becoming aware of all the other ways I criticized myself. When I ate, I criticized my food choices and the amounts I ate. Whenever I saw my reflection in a mirror or a window I made a critical comment. I tried to stop criticizing myself, but it happened so automatically I felt I was unable to control it.

Then someone suggested an alternative phrase. I liked it because it wasn't exactly positive, which felt too unreal to me, but it was better than the harsh criticism I usually doled out. The phrase was "Not bad!" I learned to say this in many situations. For example, when I unexpectedly saw my reflection in a store window, I would immediately say, "Not bad!" After completing a meal, I'd take a breath and say, sometimes aloud, "Not bad!" This was a far cry from my familiar litany of criticisms. More changes followed. I began to feel less hostile and more loving toward myself. I started to enjoy myself more and to feel more comfortable being alone. I stopped feeling full of shame and began noticing my strong points. I started to see that criticism was hurtful, not helpful. I did much better when I was nice to myself. I took better care of myself and even ate less, without any effort. I found motivation that had previously eluded me. "Not bad!" became a private joke that made me chuckle. I began to feel much better than "Not bad." In fact, I was starting to feel pretty good! And the more I praised myself, the more I behaved in ways I was proud of.

I no longer spend my days hating and criticizing myself. I speak kindly to myself, which makes me a lot more pleasant to be around!

On the next leg of your Journey, we ask you to challenge your negative thinking. We hope you will begin to notice the ways in which you speak to yourself. You may find it similar to the ways you were spoken to as a child. You may have even intensified this criticism.

Your parents may not have had options like therapy, self-help books, or support groups to help them become more loving and gentle. But you do! They also didn't have laws which made it illegal to hit a child as a form of punishment. We have these laws because we know now that children need to be treated with respect and kindness. And children aren't the only ones that need kind treatment. We all do! Any day, any moment, is a time when you can praise yourself and treat yourself in ways you always wished you had been treated. If we treated a child the way some of us treat ourselves (stuffing food into our mouths when we're not hungry, starving ourselves, forcing ourselves to exercise when we are full or ill), we could be arrested for abuse!

Suppose a child came to you and said, "I feel fat, scared, and lonely," would you say the kinds of things you say to yourself, such as, "You're a loser," "You're ugly," or even "I wish you were dead?" Would you do what you do to yourself and stuff food into her mouth, starve her when she's hungry, or force her to exercise while she's feeling so awful? Would you make her constantly focus, like you make yourself focus, on her weight, dragging her to the scale so you can berate her and make her feel worse than she already feels? This is what many of us do to ourselves. Think about a hurt child coming to you for help. Might you instead receive her with compassion and understanding? Might you show her some sympathy and honest caring? Would you possibly have her climb onto your lap and tell you about her pain? These are the ways you need to learn to treat yourself.

What would you have wanted from the adults in your life when you were a child? What do you want right now? It's up to you how you treat yourself now and how you teach others to treat you.

If you have excess weight on your body, it might be because you have been hurt and have not yet healed. It is not because you are undisciplined or lacking willpower. When you look in the mirror, it is unfair to criticize and berate yourself (you're already wounded). It would be more appropriate to look in the mirror and say to yourself, "This is my sadness I'm seeing on my body." Or, "These are my pounds of pain." Or, "I'm sorry you've been so hurt." And as you continue on your Journey, you will learn how to express your pain, rather than wear it.

Just like a muscle that's weak and out of shape, your "Praise Muscle" may be suffering from lack of use. Each time you tell yourself "You blew it," "You're so fat," or "Boy are you stupid!" you build your "Criticism Muscle." Conversely, each time you communicate something positive to yourself, like "You're making progress," "Good job," or "You're really making an effort," you are building up your "Praise Muscle." As you strengthen the "Praise Muscle," the "Criticism Muscle" weakens. Let's give it a try. Following are some exercises that you don't need a spa membership to do!

❧ *Journey One*

*Date:*_____

1. Make a list of the negative statements you regularly tell yourself:

   Make a list of the positive statements you tell yourself:

Now, starting at the bottom left of each list, draw a line up and over the top, then back down the right side, like this:

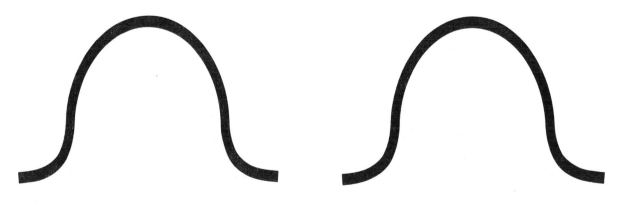

Imagine that each drawing represents a biceps muscle. Which muscle looks bigger and stronger? Challenge yourself by adding a few positive statements to the Praise Muscle right now (pump it up a little). If you have trouble doing this, ask a friend to give you some honest compliments and write them down. Just as when you are building muscle tissue, you may feel uncomfortable at first. You may cramp up or get sore. You may want to quit. Keep going. Eventually, it works. You can become happier with yourself.

2. Complete the following sentences:
   a. I'm afraid if I praise myself . . .

   _____

   _____

   _____

   _____

   b. The reasons I deserve to treat myself nicely are . . .

   _____

   _____

   _____

   _____

   _____

   c. The reasons I don't think I deserve to be treated nicely are . . .

   _____

   _____

   _____

   _____

3. Imagine a small child comes to you and tells you the same things you wrote about yourself in Question #2C.

   a. How would you respond if you were critical or abusive?

   _____

   _____

   _____

   _____

   b. How would you respond if you were loving?

   _____

   _____

   _____

   _____

c. Now try saying the loving responses to yourself. Notice how that feels. Pick one loving response and write it on several small pieces of paper. Put the notes in places where you will see them over the next few days. Every time you see one, repeat the phrase to yourself.

4. In column A, write down five "shoulds" you commonly tell yourself. In Column B, change each "should" to "could." Then add why you choose to do or not to do it.

Column A	Column B
e.g. *I should exercise today.*	*I could exercise today. I'll do it after work.*
I should call my mother.	*I could call my mother, but I'm feeling too tired, so I won't.*

5. Estimate what percentage of your time you spend criticising your body or yourself.

_____

✂ *Journey Two*

Date:_____

1. Make a list of the negative statements   Make a list of the positive
    you tell yourself on a regular basis: statements you tell yourself:

Now starting at the bottom left of each list, draw a line up and over the top, then back down the right side, like this:

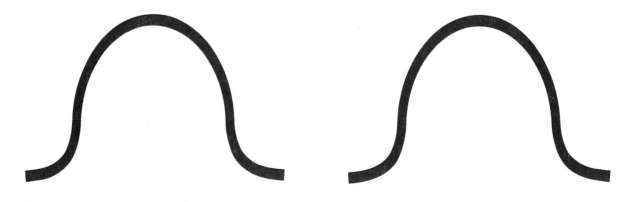

Imagine each drawing represents a biceps muscle. Which muscle looks bigger and stronger? Challenge yourself by adding a few positive statements to the Praise Muscle right now (pump it up a little). If you have trouble doing this, ask a friend to give you some honest compliments and write them down. Just as when you are building muscle tissue, you may feel uncomfortable at first. You may cramp up or get sore. Keep going. Eventually, it works.

2. Look back at Journey One, Question #1. Comparing the size of the muscles in Journey One to those you just drew, describe what you notice:

_____

_____

_____

_____

3.　　a. Write a letter to the body part you criticize the most.

Dear _____,

_____

_____

_____

_____

_____

_____

_____

_____

_____

_____

b. Now have that body part write a letter back to you.

Dear _____,

_____

_____

_____

_____

_____

_____

_____

_____

c. What did you notice? Any surprises?

_____

_____

_____

_____

_____

_____

4. The obstacles I still face when it comes to being nice to myself are . . .

_____

_____

_____

_____

_____

_____

_____

5.   a. Make a list of some great things about yourself, or some of your accomplishments:

_____

_____

_____

_____

_____

_____

b. Read the above list aloud. Read it with pride. How does it feel to praise yourself?

_____

_____

_____

_____

_____

✖ *Journey Three*

*Date:*_____

1. Make a list of the negative statements   Make a list of the positive
    you tell yourself on a regular basis: statements you tell yourself:

Now starting at the bottom left of each list, draw a line up and over the top, then back down the right side, like this:

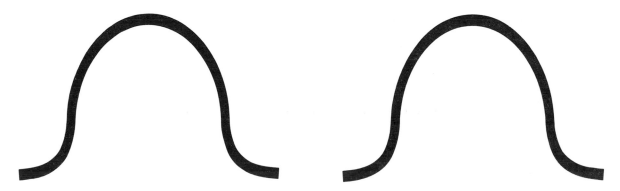

Imagine that each drawing represents a biceps muscle. Which muscle looks bigger and stronger? Challenge yourself by adding a few positive statements to the Praise Muscle right now (pump it up a little). If you have trouble doing this, ask a friend to give you some honest compliments and write them down.

2. Look back at Journeys One and Two, Question #1. Comparing the size of the muscles in the first two Journeys with the ones you just drew, write about what you notice.

_____

_____

_____

_____

3. If you were criticized as a child, where in your body do you imagine the criticisms hit? Are they still there? Draw a picture of your body, showing the stored criticisms.

4. a. What do you think would happen if you were to stop criticizing yourself?

_____

_____

_____

_____

 b. What would you have to let go of? Are you willing? Why or why not?

_____

_____

_____

_____

5. List the ways you experience "sweetness" in your life (other than food). Include the ways you give sweetness to yourself and receive it from others.

I give sweetness to myself by:	I get sweetness from others by:
Examples: *Taking hot baths* *Buying myself flowers*	*Getting massages* *Cuddling with my partner*

6. One sweet thing I could do for myself today is:

_____

_____

7. Imagine a young version of yourself. Pick any age. Now imagine your current self going up to your younger self and giving her the praise she always wanted to hear. What would you say? Write to her below.

Dear Young _____,

_____

_____

_____

_____

_____

_____

_____

Journey Four

Date:_____

1. Describe the difference between someone who loves herself and a narcissistic or conceited person.

_____

_____

_____

_____

_____

_____

2. Write a letter of praise to someone you love. (You can decide whether or not to give it.)

_____

_____

_____

_____

_____

_____

_____

3. Write a letter of praise to yourself. (Include praise for making it this far in your Journey.)

_____

_____

_____

_____

_____

_____

_____

_____

_____

4. a. What part of your body do you still criticize, and why?

_____

_____

_____

_____

_____

_____

b. How does this impact your life?

_____

_____

_____

_____

_____

c. Write a letter of apology to that body part. Include an acknowledgment for the ways in which it functions.

_____

_____

_____

_____

_____

_____

_____

_____

_____

_____

_____

_____

_____

_____

5. Write a list of non-food-related ways in which you give and get sweetness.

_____

_____

_____

_____

_____

_____

6. Look back to Journey Three, Question #5. Has your list increased? When was the last time you did one of the activities on the list?

_____

_____

7. Estimate what percentage of your time you spend criticizing yourself. Look back at Journey One, Question #5. Compare your answers and write about what you notice.

_____

_____

_____

_____

_____

8. What do you think would happen if you gave up your self-criticism and praised yourself on a regular basis?

_____

_____

_____

_____

_____

_____

Chapter 7

Black-and-White vs. Rainbow Thinking

"I can't eat this cookie! I won't eat this cookie! Oh well, maybe just one. . .
Now I blew it! I may as well eat them all and start my diet again tomorrow."

Is this a familiar scenario? Many people who suffer with food and weight problems also struggle with *Black-and-White Thinking*. This means seeing ourselves as either on or off our diet, good or bad, perfect or a failure. Black-and-White thinkers swing back and forth between two extremes. We have trouble even imagining that there could be options, compromise, or a middle ground.

We learn Black-and-White Thinking from many sources, such as our family, the dieting industry, and society. Your parents may have told you that you were "wonderful" one day, then labeled you as "bad" the next, rather than pointing out your specific strengths or weaknesses. You may have observed your mom eating excessive amounts of food one day, and starving herself the next. The dieting industry tries to convince us that eating one piece of candy will make us fat, and we get messages from our culture that if we are fat we are bad. We're left with a simplistic kind of reasoning. Good or bad. All or nothing. Always or never. Black or white. In reality, one piece of anything doesn't make anybody fat. And fat doesn't mean bad. (It may mean sad, hurt, mad, or it may be your natural body weight, but it doesn't mean bad.)

Although the motive in attempting to be at the so-called "good" extreme is to avoid the other "bad" extreme, struggling to be perfectly "good" sets us up to fail and become "bad." Depriving oneself of food eventually causes one to overeat. Excessive exercising causes burnout or injury and often leads to the inability to exercise at all. Pretending to be happy all the time and avoiding other feelings eventually leads to depression (which is often the result of pressing down your feelings). Needing to see ourselves as perfect only causes a constant feeling of inadequacy.

The most common result of perfectionism is low self-esteem. Being perfect is an impossible goal. If your objective is to be perfect — perfect eater, perfect body, perfect feelings, perfect girlfriend, perfect wife, mother, student, child — and perfection is impossible, then you have a recipe for failure.

In the early stages of healing food, weight and body issues, our Black-and-White Thinking causes difficulty because we tend to see ourselves as being either perfect or complete failures. We forget that recovery is an ongoing, ever-changing, sometimes painstakingly slow process. If we eat something we consider less than perfect, we are quick to tell ourselves, "See, this isn't working. I'll never recover." However, we guarantee that nobody (and that means nobody — okay, so we're being black-and-white!) gets into recovery and suddenly becomes a "perfect eater" (or a "perfect person").

In fact, recovery is about letting go of the need to be perfect. It's also about letting go of the idea that you're a failure. It may be hard to believe, but there is a vast array of options that lie between the black and white extremes. Taking advantage of these options involves what we call *Rainbow Thinking*. Rainbow Thinking is the alternative to Black-and-White Thinking. It means having numerous options instead of only two. It means seeing all the colors of the rainbow instead of only black and white. It means having access to all our feelings. It means accepting our humanness and imperfections and recognizing our specialness and strengths. It means believing that good enough is good enough!

Let's take a look at how Rainbow Thinking gives us more choices than Black-and-White Thinking. We used to think bread was a "bad" food and salad was a "good" food, and so we would attempt to eat a lot of salad and no bread (particularly in public!) Let's say this was the "black" in Black-and-White Thinking. And the "white" side of the equation? Having felt so deprived, we would eventually find ourselves downing a whole loaf of bread (particularly when alone). Then, feeling stuffed and ashamed, we vowed never to eat bread again (back to "black"). Until one day, one week, one month later, guess what happened? And so the cycle continued. It never occurred to us that we could have one sandwich, that we deserved to have one sandwich, that one sandwich would not make us fat. Being willing to have a sandwich instead of no bread, or a whole loaf of bread, is an example of Rainbow Thinking. Today we see Rainbow Thinking in many areas of our lives: taking a walk instead of either high-impact aerobics, or sitting on the couch; getting a few errands done instead of either compulsively doing them all, or eating instead of doing any; assertively communicating our anger to a friend instead of either raging, or saying nothing.

Just like anything new, Rainbow Thinking may be uncomfortable at first. However, after spending some time in the middle of the road getting used to being perfectly imperfect, the Journey becomes much easier and more enjoyable.

Marsea:

> *When I was offered a job in a big city, I had a challenging decision to make about my life in a small beach town. I loved where I lived, and I especially loved the converted garage I rented and had created into a beautiful home. It was a special place and held many wonderful memories of my transition into freedom from my food and weight issues. I had never been to this*

particular city and didn't really want to go there, but the job I was offered fulfilled a specific dream I had of working in an eating disorders unit in a hospital. I had never planned on leaving my current home, however, and I also knew there was no guarantee this job would work out for me. So I had to decide whether to let go of everything I loved where I was, or to let go of my dreams and stay put. All or nothing. Right? Wrong!

By this time, I had become a Rainbow Thinker. I made two Rainbow Decisions. The first was to take the job on a temporary basis — one year — with plans to move back when the year was up, unless, of course, I wanted to stay longer (which was what happened). The second decision was to hold on to my studio by subletting it while I was gone. This ended up working well for a friend who needed a long-term temporary place to live.

As it turned out, I spent three years in the new city. During that time, I became secure enough to let go of my studio, trusting I'd be able to find a nice place to live when I returned (which I did). Interestingly, the landlord of the studio offered it to me again when I returned because he liked me and admired how I had handled my dilemma. Rainbow Thinking has taught me how to live creatively. As a result, my life is colorfully full of options!

An important first step in changing Black-and-White Thinking is to notice when you're doing it. Of course, if you have Black-and-White Thinking, you probably believe that simply noticing isn't enough! But noticing is somewhere in between being unaware and completely stopping the behavior. Becoming aware, without criticizing ourselves, is part of the rainbow. For most of us, it's much easier to be gentle and flexible with other people than with ourselves, so this step of accepting yourself while paying attention to black-and-white thought patterns is an important one. Remember: **Nothing positive comes from treating yourself negatively!**

Commonly we ask our clients what expectations they have. Upon hearing their lists: "Thin by May 1st," "Exercise two hours daily," "Eliminate all sugar and fat from my diet," we tell them it's no wonder they are exhausted, not reaching their goals, and feeling like failures. Their goals are the product of Black-and-White Thinking.

Rather than trying again to accomplish what you've been unable to do for years (i.e. diet and keep the weight off, or be perfect at anything) why not try to change your unrealistic (and often cruel) expectations, and instead create goals that are loving and attainable? Dare to be average!

❧ *Journey One*

Date:_____

1. Write about some of the ways you learned to have Black-and-White Thinking.

> *Examples:*
> *Mom was always either really happy or really mad.*
> *My teacher gave me an award one day, ignored me the next.*

_____

_____

_____

_____

_____

2.   a. Add to the Black and White columns below your extreme expectations and behaviors. Cover any or all areas of your life (including work, family, play, chores).

BLACK	WHITE
Examples:	
I can't have any fat grams today.	*Forget it, I'll just binge on everything.*
I will exercise every day this week.	*I'll just end up staying home and watching TV, vowing to run three miles the next day.*
I should answer every question in this book.	*I don't answer any.*

b. In the Black-and-White columns below, transfer your lists from above. Then, practicing Rainbow Thinking, create some alternatives that lie in between the extremes, and put these in the Rainbow column. Remember: Rainbow Thinking is realistic, flexible, and gentle.

BLACK	RAINBOW	WHITE
No bread.	I can have a sandwich today.	Binge on bread.
No fat.	I can listen to my body and eat moderately. I will pay attention to whether my cravings are physical or emotional.	Binge on junk food.
Exercise daily.	I'll exercise 3 times this week. I can walk instead of jog if I feel like it.	Sit on couch; hate myself.
Answer all questions in workbook.	I'll answer the questions I feel like answering.	I won't answer any; what's the use?

3.   a. Now let's do a little stretching exercise: Think about a problem in your life that is causing you stress. It could be with work, your weight, another person; any area. Write down some of the ways you tell yourself you "should" be handling this situation.

_____

_____

_____

_____

_____

_____

b. Now here comes the stretching part: Using Rainbow Thinking, come up with at least 10 other options for handling the situation. Include some funny and outrageous options.

e.g. *THE PROBLEM: I went on a date and the guy hasn't called me since. My BLACK-AND-WHITE SOLUTION: Tell myself that maybe I'm not pretty enough or thin enough for him and I'll never have a boyfriend.*

RAINBOW OPTIONS:

1. Assume he must have lost my number, and call him.

2. Call a girlfriend for support.

3. Decide I didn't like him anyway.

4. Write him a note thanking him for a good time.

5. Crawl under the covers and don't come out for a week.

6. Call and angrily ask him why he hasn't called.

7. Go out with his best friend.

8. Realize he may not have been right for me and that's okay.

9. Make plans for how I can meet other guys.

10. _____

(See what you can come up with)

Now, you try it:

THE PROBLEM:

_____

_____

_____

_____

MY BLACK-AND-WHITE-SOLUTION:

_____

_____

_____

_____

RAINBOW OPTIONS: (Be creative! Include funny and outrageous options; they help you stretch!)

1. _____

2. _____

3. _____

4. _____

5. _____

6. _____

7. _____

8. _____

9. _____

10. _____

This sign designates what we will call a Spontaneous Road Trip. A Spontaneous Road Trip is akin to deciding to go off the beaten path and explore unknown territory. When you arrive at this sign in your workbook, we encourage you to do whatever you want on this page. You can use it to express anything going on for you at this time. You can draw, write spontaneously about your thoughts and feelings, make a collage, write a poem, insert a photograph of yourself... anything that will help you explore and record this current part of your Journey. (Remember there is no right or wrong way to do this!)

❧ *Journey Two*

*Date:*_____

1. Get to know the perfectionist in you (use your imagination here):
   a. What does she look like?

   _____

   _____

   b. How old is she?

   _____

   _____

   c. What does she say to you?

   _____

   _____

   d. Who does her voice sound like and of whom does she remind you?

   _____

   _____

   e. Give her a name:

   _____

   _____

   f. What do you want her to know right now?

   _____

   _____

   g. How does she respond?

   _____

   _____

   h. How do you answer her?

   _____

   _____

2. Describe someone you know who is an example of a Rainbow Thinker. (If you don't know anyone, make up someone and give him/her a name.)

   _____

   _____

   _____

3. Describe a scenario in which you tend to use (or think you use) Black-and-White Thinking.

For example: When I go to parties, I am either on a strict diet or I completely stuff myself, thinking I'll start over again tomorrow.

_____

_____

_____

_____

_____

_____

_____

_____

4. Now, using the same example, create a new scene using Rainbow Thinking.

For example: When going to a party, I can plan on eating a moderate amount of what ever is available even if some of it is what I consider to be fattening." If I feel myself losing control, I will call a supportive friend.

(Note: If you can't think of any new options, ask yourself what the person from Question #2 would say.)

_____

_____

_____

_____

_____

_____

_____

_____

❧ *Journey Three*

*Date:*_____

1. a. Think of some times as a young person when you tried to play a sport or creative activity and you thought you didn't do it right, well enough, or perfectly. What did you decide then about yourself or the activity?

For example: I didn't have a date for my high school prom. This confirmed that, indeed, I was unlovable.

_____

_____

_____

_____

_____

_____

b. What new decision would you like to make and hold on to at this point?

For example: I am lovable, even though I didn't have a date for my prom.

_____

_____

_____

_____

_____

2. Make a list of some areas in which you are still experiencing Black-and-White Thinking.

_____

_____

_____

_____

_____

_____

3. Referring back to Journey One, describe areas in which your thinking has changed, and areas in which it has not.

_____

_____

_____

4. Pick a situation or a belief that feels totally black or white to you.

    a. Write it down, along with the only solutions you can think of:

    _____

    _____

    _____

    _____

    _____

    b. See if you can come up with at least three other options. Be creative!

    1. _____

    2. _____

    3. _____

    c. Ask someone close to you for three additional options.

    1. _____

    2. _____

    3. _____

5. What do you think would happen if you practiced Rainbow Thinking on a regular basis?

_____

_____

_____

🌿 *Journey Four*

*Date:*_____

1. What do you think would happen if you let go of the need to be perfect?

_____

_____

_____

_____

_____

2. In what areas are you still thinking in black-and-white terms?

_____

_____

_____

_____

_____

3.   a. Pick one situation that you are struggling with and write down the two main (black-and-white) options you have in your mind.

_____

_____

_____

_____

b. What feelings are you aware of in your body when you think about these options?

_____

_____

_____

_____

4. a. Expand your thinking by coming up with 5 additional options. Get creative!

1.

_____

2.

_____

3.

_____

4.

_____

5.

_____

b. What feelings are you aware of as you think about these new options?

_____

_____

_____

_____

5. Review Journey Three, Question #4. What happened with the situation you wrote about?

_____

_____

_____

_____

_____

6. In what areas have you let go of the need to be perfect? How has that affected your life?

_____

_____

_____

_____

_____

Chapter 8

The Binge/Deprive Cycle vs. Loving Limits

We live in a society that caters to our desire for immediate gratification. Instant oats, instant coffee, instant potatoes. One-hour photos, one-hour eyeglasses, one- day liposuction. It's no wonder we feel the need to instantly feed our hunger when we want food, or immediately squelch a need or a feeling when one surfaces.

Paradoxically, this same society tells us to eat less — less fat, calories, and sweets. We're told to enjoy all the "goodies" as fast as we can, and then warned against eating those very same foods. Open up any women's magazine. It is common to see Betty Crocker's thick, moist, chocolate cake on one page, and Nordic Track's revolutionary cross-country climber on the next. Eat more, weigh less. Hurry up, slow down. Buy more, save more. Confused yet?

If instant gratification (eating whatever you want whenever you want) is on one end of the spectrum, and deprivation (not allowing yourself to eat what or when you want) is on the other end, then *Loving Limits* is somewhere in between. Loving Limits is both giving yourself what you want and maintaining limits. Unlike a diet, where someone else tells you what to eat, with Loving Limits you utilize your intimate knowledge of yourself (which will grow over time) in combination with feedback and support from those who understand this recovery process. Loving Limits helps you make daily choices about what and what not to eat.

A 500-calorie a day diet certainly entails limits, but it is not loving. Exercising regularly is a healthy goal, but doing it when you are sick, injured, or exhausted is not loving. Losing 20 pounds through strict dieting may help you achieve the weight loss you wanted, but your unloving methods will likely cause you to rebel, eat more, continue your self-hating behavior, and regain the weight. Weight loss achieved without self-love is, at best, short-lived.

On the other hand, some people rid themselves of all structure and limits, claiming they have tried their last diet and won't restrict themselves again. They resolve to love themselves no matter what and eat whatever they want. For some, this is the solution. For others, the absence of guidelines causes them to eat uncontrollably, thus feeling more disconnected from themselves than ever.

After years of dieting and/or bingeing, many people find it difficult to know when and how to limit themselves. Sometimes we forget (or don't even know) that we are recovering from dieting and diet mentality as well as overeating. We become too rigid with our limits or are afraid to have any at all. Generally, people who have had a lot of rigidity in their eating need to learn how to loosen up their limits, and people who have eaten without restraint need to learn how to set some. We had one client who spent years counting calories and avoiding fats. Her recovery entailed learning how to eat desserts moderately and to get support in dealing with the fears that arose when she did. Another client never set any food limits. She grazed on food and coffee drinks all day long. For her, recovery meant learning to say a loving "no" to herself when, in her heart, she knew she was eating or drinking compulsively.

While the specifics of each person's food and weight issues differ, most disordered eaters tend to judge food in terms of "good" or "bad" as a way of trying to set limits (i.e. Do eat salad. Don't eat cake.). Because this type of thinking is so much a part of the diet mentality that helped *create* your problems, we suggest that you begin to adopt a new line of thinking. Try asking yourself the following three questions before you eat this week: 1. What does the dieter in me think I should eat? 2. What does the overeater in me want to eat? 3. What does my heart say?

Although it may take several months before you can actually begin to hear and act on what your heart says, the experience of asking yourself these important questions will help you gain clarity on what is right for you to eat and not eat.

In the early stages of recovery, you may have difficulty knowing what is best for you because you have been inundated with myths from the diet industry about what you "should" and "should not" eat. Most of us have taken these "rules" to heart, and our hearts are confused about how to guide us. Here are some alternative guidelines that can help you distinguish between loving reasons to eat and self-destructive reasons to eat:

Loving Reasons to Eat:
Physical Hunger
Nutrition
Convenience
Pleasure

Self-Destructive Reasons to Eat:
Guilt
Anger
Shame
Loneliness
Anxiety
Feeling full
Boredom
Excitement
Other:

The loving reasons to eat are surprising to many people, so we will explain:

Physical Hunger seems like an obvious loving reason to eat, but many of us ignore our hunger even though its purpose is to tell us when our bodies need food. People with weight issues, especially those who have frequently dieted, tend to mistrust their hunger and do not regard it as important information. (Some people never even let themselves get to the point of feeling physically hungry.) Learning to distinguish between physical and emotional hunger, the subject of the next chapter, will help you become clearer about when you are physically hungry and needing to eat.

Nutrition refers to eating the specific foods our body needs at any given time, like oranges when we have a cold, or protein if we're experiencing low energy, or a salad after a few days with no vegetables. If we pay attention to our body's signals, we'll sense when we need a specific type of food for our body's proper functioning.

Convenience is about the fact that most of us lead very busy lives and don't always have the time to plan and eat our meals according to our body's schedule. For example, if you know you are going to have to wait many hours before your next opportunity to eat, it might be appropriate to eat something even if you are not yet hungry. Sometimes, for convenience, we need to let it be okay that we're not eating the healthiest of meals. If you don't have time in a busy day to prepare a healthy meal, it may work best to eat prepared foods. Many of us with food and weight issues get so anxious when we cannot eat "perfectly" that we end up overeating or even bingeing over an "imperfect" meal or a food we think we shouldn't have eaten. Some of us have been so rigid and inflexible that we have avoided social situations because we couldn't eat "perfectly," and that became more important to us than the socializing. With Rainbow Thinking and Loving Limits, this no longer needs to happen. We no longer have to obsess on food so that it robs us of life and relationships. We learn that, for the sake of convenience, we can be flexible at times about when or what we eat.

The final loving reason to eat is for **pleasure**. Just because we have food or weight issues does not mean we have to give up receiving pleasure from food! In fact, it is important that we do enjoy our food and eat foods we enjoy. It is perfectly okay to eat foods you love, as long as you can eat them lovingly.

If your relationship with a particular food is so charged that you cannot eat it lovingly or in moderation, then, for a time, the loving action may be to forego it. Just remember that as you heal your food issues, you can get to a point where that food becomes safe to eat again. Refraining from eating a certain food is only temporary; it is a way to love yourself, not to punish yourself.

Most of the self-destructive reasons to eat have to do with using food to alter your emotions. When you eat to numb or change feelings, you end up feeling out of control and causing harm to your body. The more loving response may be to refrain from eating when you sense you're trying to suppress your emotions. By refraining from eating at those times, you will be giving yourself the opportunity to learn healthier ways of coping. You have an opportunity to release and heal your feelings, rather than medicating them by eating instead. If you can't come up with any alternatives to eating, you can call a safe person. Talk to this person about your feelings and ask for suggestions of appropriate ways to respond to them. When you are upset or bored or angry or anxious, it is not appropriate to turn to food for support.

It is appropriate to turn to safe people.

Loving Limits is about honesty, willingness and courage. It takes rigorous honesty to know what is right for you to eat at any given moment (and right may include a cookie!) It takes willingness to then do what you know is right, and it takes courage to be present for your feelings and your relationships.

Loving Limits includes recognizing when you are using food unlovingly, and finding out what it is you are truly hungry for. It also means recognizing when you are depriving yourself and figuring out what you really want to eat. While many of us think our problem is overeating, we tend to become undereaters quite easily. Undereating is as unloving as overeating and is a setup for a binge. Undernourishment compromises our physical health and diminishes our intellectual abilities. Loving Limits means that we eat regularly, whether we are upset, depressed or high on life.

Marsea:

For many years Binge/Deprive was my lifestyle. I called it "Bad Days" and "Good Days." If I starved myself or ate only diet-type foods, it was a "good day." If I ate one thing I considered "bad," the whole day was ruined. Once that happened, I would go into "bad day" mode and eat, non-stop, everything I normally forbade myself to eat.

This behavior was encouraged by my grandmother who, concerned about her weight, discovered a diet that prescribed drinking special shakes every other day and eating "regularly" on alternate days. My grandmother and I followed this diet as if it were a recreational activity. We went shopping together for the shake ingredients, discussed what foods we'd eat on our eating days, forecasted our weight loss, and commiserated about our hunger and our weight problems. We loved this diet. On alternate days, when we were allowed to eat, we let ourselves have whatever we wanted. That made the days without food seem tolerable. The only problem was this: we weren't losing any weight! (Yet we kept trying — this diet was guaranteed!)

It seems ludicrous to me today, but at the time I honestly believed that I could eat normally every other day and that I would lose weight, even though I was starving and obsessed with food. This diet fit right into my already solid belief that deprivation was necessary and that "next time" I wouldn't binge. I didn't know then that deprivation was a part of my eating disorder, that bingeing and depriving myself were two sides of the same coin. One led to the other, and "good" and "bad" were both part of a faulty belief system.

Much later I realized that in order to move from the Binge/Deprive Cycle to the moderation of Loving Limits, I had to acknowledge that deprivation was as much a part of my problem as bingeing. This was hard, and scary, to do. I had always seen deprivation as a good thing. To let go of it was to risk losing control. It also meant letting go of this particular bond with my grandmother (and other women I knew who also deprived themselves of food). Eventually I began to see that "control" was an illusion. None of the women I knew who were "controlling" their weight, were actually in control; in fact, their weight continued to climb. I came to realize that all my efforts at control had led to nothing but weight gain and a profound feeling of failure. My only hope was to try a new way.

I let go of deprivation. I started allowing myself to eat. I gave myself the same permission to eat that thin people seemed to give themselves. In the beginning, it was terrifying. Certain foods were very difficult to eat in moderation — I didn't want to stop. I had to learn to say to myself, "That's enough for now, Sweetie. You can have more later." I stopped telling myself, "You can never eat that again!" I stopped telling myself that one instance of overeating had ruined my day.

In terms of Loving Limits, after some trial and error, I made a decision to confine my eating to meal times. This decision came from a sincere desire to make my life easier, not as a form of dieting or method of weight loss. Though I was no longer depriving myself of food, I also didn't want to think about food all the time. I found that the structure of three meals a day was comfortable and plentiful for me. It was helpful for me to stay within that structure because it relieved me of thinking about food in between meals. Again, it was not about deprivation or dieting; it was about ease, convenience, and the reassurance that I would, indeed, have another opportunity to eat again soon. So, every day, I had a breakfast, a lunch, and a dinner.

Over and over, day after day, I reassured myself that I could eat whatever I wanted at my next meal. And that there would be another meal after that. After so many years of deprivation, I needed a lot of reassurance and time to begin to trust myself. Every day, over and over, I had to prove to myself that I was free to eat whatever I wanted, within my chosen loving structure. And as I did this, I found less and less need to binge. At first, I stuck to my structure quite rigidly, afraid that eating snacks would set off a binge. But as I began to trust myself (and deal with my unresolved pain) my meals got calmer and saner. I began to know when I was physically hungry, and I began to trust myself with snacks when my body needed them. Eventually I was able to let go of the structured meals and to eat when I was hungry — sometimes two meals, sometimes three, sometimes four. Whatever was most loving for me that day.

I no longer feel out of control, and I no longer have the desire to deprive myself. Consequently, I no longer feel a need to binge. Most of the time, I eat moderate, loving meals. If I do eat too much (which, by the way, even "normal" eaters periodically do) I follow three rules: Don't Panic, Don't Binge, and Don't Diet. Then, eventually, I digest my food and become comfortable again.

Loving Limits is not only about establishing limits with food. We need limits in all areas of our lives. We may overeat or undereat to avoid the discomfort we feel when other people make us angry. Sometimes our weight is a nonverbal attempt to set limits when we cannot trust ourselves to set limits verbally.

Sue, for example, was out of control with her eating and her weight when she came to us for help. As a result of learning to identify her feelings, she is now more aware when somebody does something she doesn't like. Because she no longer stuffs her feelings down with food, she finds opportunities to express her limits when she needs to do so. Week after week, she reported her success stories about being honest with people. When her hairdresser advised her to try a new diet, Sue said, "That hurts my feelings." When her niece bad-mouthed Sue's sister, Sue told her, "I don't like it when you talk like that." After years of criticism from her daughter, Sue finally told her, "It hurts me when you call me 'fat' and I don't want you to do that anymore." Interestingly, her daughter was surprised that her remarks about mother's weight bothered her. Because of Sue's silence in the past, her daughter thought she didn't care.

In the past, Sue ignored her own feelings and needs because she didn't want to "rock the boat." She didn't think her own feelings mattered and she believed that other people's feelings were all important. Sue had no idea that her inability to set limits related to her problem with overeating and her inability to lose weight.

When we neglect to set limits with people, we end up feeling resentful or hurt, and then we overeat, undereat or purge. Loving Limits means finding kind and compassionate ways to say "No," "Stop," or "That won't work for me."

We believe that within each of us exists a part that knows the truth — a part that knows when we just said "yes" and we really meant "no," a part that knows when we've had enough to eat or when we need more. Some call this their intuition. Some call it their gut, their heart, or their instinct. Some call it their Higher Power or God. We refer to it as "the part of you that knows." Right now that part may be a stranger to you. It may have been so stuffed, ignored, or silenced that even you cannot find it. The more you pay attention, however, the clearer it will become.

The following exercises will help you learn how to begin to think in terms of Loving Limits, rather than bouncing back and forth between excess and deprivation.

🌿 *Journey One*

Date:_____

1. List below the ways in which you deprive yourself.

For example: "I won't eat any sweet foods."

_____

_____

_____

_____

_____

_____

_____

_____

2. Now list what you imagine happens to you when you relinquish all limits.

For example: "I would eat everything I was depriving myself of."

_____

_____

_____

_____

_____

_____

_____

_____

_____

_____

3. Now let's explore what an attitude of Loving Limits would sound like.
   Here are some real-life examples:

"I don't want to go to the dentist today, but I need to go once a year."
"I try to exercise 3 times a week, but my foot hurts; I need to rest it."
"I don't feel like exercising today, but I know I'll feel better if I do."
"I'm still hungry; I think I'll have another serving."
"I want another serving, but I know I'm not physically hungry. I think I'm anxious about work and I need to let myself feel it."

Create some of your own examples:

_____
_____
_____
_____
_____
_____

4. Ask yourself the following three questions:

   a. What does the dieter in me think I should eat today?

   _____
   _____
   _____

   b. What does the overeater in me want to eat today?

   _____
   _____
   _____

   c. What does my heart say?

   _____
   _____
   _____

5. In this next exercise, create a dialogue. Write it as if it is a conversation between two voices. One voice will be you, and the other will be a loving voice ("the part of you that knows," a loving parent or grandparent, an angel, an animal, a special friend . . .).

Here are some ideas to begin your dialogue:

Ask the loving voice what it thinks of you. Or tell it what you think of yourself. Ask it how you could get to know it better or what it thinks you could do to heal from your food and weight issues. Then let the loving voice respond. Continue dialoguing for as long as you like. Remember, this is a new relationship, so it's okay if it's awkward at first. If you can't think of anything right away, sit quietly until the words come.

Me: _____

_____

Loving Voice (L.V.): _____

_____

Me: _____

_____

L.V.: _____

_____

Me: _____

_____

L.V.: _____

_____

Me: _____

_____

L.V.: _____

_____

6. Make a list of goals and expectations you would like to have, using an attitude of Loving Limits. (If you get stuck, ask that loving voice from Question #5 for help.)

_____

_____

_____

_____

_____

_____

_____

7. Read over your above goals and expectations. Are they loving? Do they provide gentle guidelines? Anything you'd like to change or add?

_____

_____

_____

_____

_____

_____

_____

8. What is one thing "the part of you that knows" wants to say to you right now?

_____

_____

_____

_____

_____

_____

_____

_____

_____

❦ *Journey Two*

Date:_____

1. List below the ways in which you limit yourself. Are they loving or unloving? Are they helpful or hurtful?

_____

_____

_____

_____

2.   a. Referring to the list above, from where did each of these ideas come?

_____

_____

_____

_____

        b. Which ones feel right for you to keep; which would you like to discard?

_____

_____

_____

_____

3. In this next exercise, create a dialogue between two parts of yourself. One part is your critical voice, the voice that tells you you're not o.k. (You know the one!) The other part is your loving voice. (This voice may still be hard to hear.) Write as if these two parts are having a conversation.

Here is a brief example of a dialogue:

Critical Voice (C.V.): You should have lost more weight by now!

Loving Voice (L.V.): My approach to losing weight makes more sense now, and I'm changing at a pace I feel comfortable with. Besides, every time I've lost weight quickly, I've gained it back.

C.V.: But I can't stand how you look.

L.V.: It hurts me so much when you say things like that. Plus, it makes me want to eat more. I have put on weight because of my pain, not because I am "bad."

Begin writing your own dialogue; continue as long as you like:

Critical Voice: _____

_____

Loving Voice: _____

_____

C.V.: _____

_____

L.V.: _____

_____

C.V.: _____

_____

L.V.: _____

_____

C.V.: _____

_____

L.V.: _____

_____

4. Reread the above dialogue. Who does the critical voice remind you of? What does is it feel like to read it?

_____

_____

_____

_____

_____

_____

_____

5   a. What are some ways you could respond to your critical voice other than believing it?
Examples: talking back to it, shaking your head no, laughing at it, telling a safe person.

_____

_____

_____

b. If you talked back to it, what would you say?

_____

_____

_____

6. What does the "part of you that knows" want to say to you right now?

_____

_____

_____

7.   a. With whom do you currently need to set limits?

_____

_____

b. About what do you need to set limits?

_____

_____

_____

c. Imagine you were lovingly telling this person your limits. What would you say?

_____

_____

_____

This sign designates what we will call a Spontaneous Road Trip. A Spontaneous Road Trip is akin to deciding to go off the beaten path and explore unknown territory. When you arrive at this sign in your workbook, we encourage you to do whatever you want on this page. You can use it to express anything going on for you at this time. You can draw, write spontaneously about your thoughts and feelings, make a collage, write a poem, insert a photograph of yourself . . . anything that will help you explore and record this current part of your Journey. (Remember there is no right or wrong way to do this!)

❧ *Journey Three*

Date:_____

1. In this next exercise you will create a dialogue between two parts of yourself. One part is your critical voice, the voice that tells you you're not o.k. (you know the one!) The other part is your loving voice (this voice may still be hard to hear). Write as if these two parts are having a conversation.

Here is a brief example of a dialogue:

Critical Voice (C.V.): You should have lost more weight by now!

Loving Voice (L.V.): My approach to losing weight makes more sense now, and I'm changing at a pace I feel comfortable with. Besides, every time I've lost weight quickly, I've gained it back.

C.V.: But I can't stand how you look.

L.V.: It hurts me so much when you say things like that. Plus, it makes me want to eat more.

C.V.: I am just trying to help you. You look horrible, and it makes me sad to see you so fat.

L.V.: You are not helping. I'd rather we talked about the sadness than have you criticize my body all the time.

Begin writing your own dialogue; continue as long as you like:

Critical Voice: _____

_____

Loving Voice: _____

_____

C.V.: _____

_____

L.V.: _____

_____

C.V.: _____

_____

L.V.: _____

_____

C.V. _____

_____

L.V. _____

_____

2. Referring back to Journey One and Two (Question #1), make a list of old rules and former methods of depriving yourself that you have let go of. Has anything uncomfortable happened to you as a result? Has anything positive happened?

_____

_____

_____

_____

_____

_____

3. What feelings did your deprivation mask and distract you from?

_____

_____

_____

_____

_____

4. Write about some of the ways you have become more loving with yourself since you began this workbook. How has this changed you?

_____

_____

_____

_____

_____

_____

_____

_____

_____

_____

_____

5. What are your goals now in terms of Loving Limits? What harshness do you want to let go of now? What loving structure do you want to instill?

_____

_____

_____

_____

_____

_____

_____

_____

_____

_____

_____

_____

❧ *Journey Four*

*Date:*_____

1. Describe the difference between Loving Limits and diet mentality.

_____

_____

_____

_____

_____

_____

_____

_____

2. List below three times you have used Loving Limits. What did you say to yourself?

_____

_____

_____

_____

_____

_____

3. Given the three instances above, how would you have handled each in the past?

_____

_____

_____

_____

_____

_____

4. Write about the last time you were in the Binge/Deprive Cycle. What self-hating statements did you say to yourself?

_____

_____

_____

_____

_____

_____

_____

_____

5. What would have been a different way to handle that experience using Loving Limits?

_____

_____

_____

_____

_____

_____

_____

_____

6. What feelings surface when you think of truly loving yourself?

_____

_____

_____

_____

_____

_____

_____

_____

7. What does the "part of you that knows" want to say to you right now?

_____

_____

_____

_____

_____

_____

_____

8. What feelings do you notice when you connect with the "part of you that knows?"

_____

_____

_____

_____

_____

_____

_____

Chapter 9

Emotional vs. Physical Hunger

Many people with food and weight problems have difficulty distinguishing between their emotional hunger and their physical hunger. After all, if you've turned to food to handle your emotions in the past, it may now be hard to know whether you're feeling physically hungry or feeling angry, sad, lonely or anxious. If you find yourself heading toward the refrigerator, you may indeed be hungry for food, but you could also be starving for attention, craving human comfort, or filled with intolerable emotions.

Physical hunger is when your body needs nourishment. Emotional hunger is when your soul needs nourishment. This leg of the Journey is about learning to distinguish between the two. Let's explore how we learned to get physical hunger and emotional hunger mixed up in the first place.

Many families have rituals that dictate when we should or shouldn't be hungry. For example, if the family dinner is at 6 p.m. and you come home hungry at 5 p.m, you may have been told you would "spoil your appetite" if you ate any earlier. On the other hand, if you weren't hungry for dinner at 6 p.m., your parents may have insisted that you "finish everything on your plate" anyway. These rules teach us to ignore our body's signals.

One important reason for the family meal is for members to have time to connect with each other. However, if a family member is not hungry at a designated meal and is forced or pressured into eating, the last thing they will feel is "connected." Many of us grow up accustomed to eating when we're not hungry and never learn that there are other ways of connecting with people, aside from eating.

Another reason we get our hungers mixed up is a general misunderstanding about the function of emotions. When we were young, our parents, or other adults, (often with the best intentions) may have tried to comfort us with food when we were feeling upset. What we really needed then was to feel our feelings. Feeding children food to curb their feelings interrupts this necessary, natural process. It also trains us to suppress our feelings with food so that, as adults, we eat when we're upset rather than dealing with what's causing us to be upset. Then, as parents, we tend to quiet our own children's feelings by offering them food, instead of encouraging them to feel by listening to them, holding them, or simply letting them be. Until you begin to tolerate your own feelings, you won't feel comfortable tolerating your children's or anyone else's feelings, and the cycle will continue.

Often, we don't even recognize that we are having feelings; we think we just feel "hungry." For example, you might be angry at work but, believing you are hungry, you go into the staff lounge and eat several donuts. You could be bored, lonely, tired, or even thirsty at the end of your day; thinking you are hungry, you turn to food. At this point in your life, your hunger, overeating or need to control food may be the only indicator that something is wrong. You may claim to "feel fine" emotionally, but this is because you aren't really experiencing, or are unaware of, your feelings. (We like to tell our clients that the word "fine" stands for Frustrated, Insecure, Neurotic and Emotional!)

Our culture gives us many confusing messages about physical hunger and food. On the one hand, there are numerous occasions — business lunches, birthday parties, dinner parties, or holiday gatherings — when we are expected to eat, even if we're not necessarily hungry. On the other hand, we are encouraged to starve ourselves, deprive ourselves, and not eat when we are hungry in order to achieve a perfect body. Despite the fact that regular, balanced meals are necessary for our body's proper functioning and overall well-being, we see countless clients who not only skip meals, but often don't eat all day.

We once had a coworker who was an incredible role model in terms of listening to her body. We often joked that she must have come from another planet, as she did not act like any other woman we knew when it came to food and weight. She was at her natural weight, and she felt good about her body. She ate whenever she was physically hungry (and we mean whenever!) and did not eat when she wasn't hungry. We were amazed! We have seen her eating a pop tart in line at the post office, and we have also seen her have only tea at a staff luncheon because she wasn't hungry. Her eating and not eating had nothing to do with other people (pleasing them or insulting them). Her eating had to do with her body's pleasure and physical needs. (P.S. She did say she was, indeed, from Planet Earth!)

Our culture also gives us confusing messages about feelings and food. Just look at the world of advertising. A number of product campaigns try to sell us on the notion that their sweet cereal, chocolate coffee, or rich ice cream will energize us, soothe us, cheer us up, or reward us after a hard day. And we buy it!

You may be wondering, "How do I distinguish between emotional and physical hunger?" One indicator that you may be emotionally hungry rather than physically hungry is that you eat and eat and never feel full. When you do this, you not only continue to have the unresolved emotions, but you take on additional problems as well, such as feeling ashamed, alone, stuffed and physically ill. Also, if you eat when you are not physically hungry to begin with, you will not attain an appropriate feeling of fullness or receive a signal to stop.

Another clue that you may be emotionally hungry is that you crave certain types of foods. We tend to gravitate toward specific textures of foods when we have certain unmet emotional needs. For example, soft and/or creamy foods may indicate a need for comfort. Many people binge on ice cream, muffins, pudding, or noodles when they feel lonely, hurt or sad. We tend to eat hard, crunchy foods when we are angry and have a need to discharge energy by gnawing and crunching. Chips, popcorn, crackers, cookies and pretzels fall into this category. Many of us also binge on foods that our parents seemed to be comforted by, or foods that we were "comforted" with as children. If mom made you noodles when you were sick, you may find yourself turning to noodles when you are emotionally, not physically, hungry. Certain foods may represent a certain person for you, and when you have an unresolved problem with that person, you may turn to the food that corresponds, in your mind, to that person.

Linda, a client of ours, used to find herself making and bingeing on her mother's special cake recipe when she was angry with her mother. This happened unconsciously, and while she was doing it she had no idea why. Her anger got turned in on herself when she couldn't express it to her mother. The whole time she was making and eating this cake, she was berating herself and hating herself for doing it, completely unaware of her unexpressed anger toward her mother.

Indicators that you are physically hungry can be: low energy level, feeling empty, some irritability, stomach rumbling, or mouth watering. But remember, these symptoms of hunger differ for everyone, and when we really want to eat (for emotional reasons) we are capable of manufacturing them. The best way you can tell if you are physically hungry is to ask the "part of you that knows."

As you learn to feed your emotional hungers in ways other than food, you'll begin to know when you're physically hungry. You'll eat what you need, and will be satisfied with the right amount.

There is no food that will fill emotional hunger and no diet that will curb it. When you are emotionally hungry, you need to tend to your emotions. When you are physically hungry, you need to eat food. You are the only one who can know the nature of your hunger.

Andrea:

> *I recently experienced a great example of distinguishing between emotional and physical hunger. I was at a meeting with a large number of people in the room. I was one of the presenters and would be speaking in the next 5-10 minutes. I began to feel very scared about it. I developed butterflies in my stomach and sweaty palms. I tried to ignore the feelings by focusing on the announcements that were being given, and the fear seemed to dissipate. The next thought I had was of food. I remember thinking I was "starving" all of a sudden. I was surprised at how quickly it had come on, particularly because I had just had breakfast before arriving at the meeting. Then I realized that my stomach was tight because I was scared. I was mistaking the trembling and tension in my stomach for hunger because it was easier (and more automatic) to think about food than to feel my fear. A simple, honest mistake. It can happen to anyone, right? The good news is that this all took place within a few minutes, and I had the awareness to sit with it and think it through. (The commitment to speak definitely helped me stay in the room!) In the past, I would have been eating before I ever realized what I was feeling, and why.*

At any given moment, underneath all your "shoulds," rules and judgments, there is a "part of you that knows" what you are truly hungry for, whether it's broccoli, cake or a hug. There are a variety of ways to determine exactly what it is you are hungry for. For starters, pay close attention to your feelings. This week, before eating, try asking yourself, "Am I physically or emotionally hungry right now?" If you don't know, notice that. Ask yourself again at the next opportunity. For now, you don't necessarily need to change anything about your eating habits. By simply noticing and labeling your hungers, you're taking an important step.

Another way to distinguish between the two kinds of hungers is to discuss your eating and your feelings with a person you trust, preferably someone who understands the recovery process. On our personal Journeys, we have frequently called each other to discuss our feelings and confusion in this process. There would be times when we knew we had eaten or wanted to eat even though we weren't physically hungry. At the same time, we had no idea what kinds of feelings we were suppressing. It wasn't easy to make these calls to each other, but we were motivated by the emotional pain and humiliation of bingeing. At first, we couldn't imagine how talking to someone could possibly help our eating problem, but we knew we couldn't get through the confusion alone. Eventually we could see that reaching out had a profound effect on our eating. Through making phone calls in our vulnerable moments, we learned how to identify our feelings, express our feelings, get reassurance and direction, and develop intimacy with another person.

Many of our clients are afraid to make outreach calls because they don't know what to say. Here are some of the words we suggest to help them get started:

"Hi, I don't know what's going on with me, but I think I need support because all I want to do is eat, yet I know I'm not physically hungry."

Or, *"I have no idea what's going on, I just know I feel fat. Can you talk or listen for a little while?"*

Or, *"Hi. This is really scary for me, but I wanted to try calling someone instead of eating right now."*

Or, *"Are you available to talk right now? I've been eating all day and I want to stop. I have no idea what's really going on for me. If you're busy, I'll definitely keep calling people until I find someone who is available, but I thought I'd try you first."*

People in our support groups who take the risk to call other group members begin to notice profound changes in their eating. Their progress underscores the importance of breaking isolation. When we are alone, we are more likely to get into the thinking patterns that lead us to overeat or obsess about our bodies. When we reach out, we break those patterns.

Sometimes we are afraid to reach out to others because we don't know what we would do if someone called us. When people reach out to you, remember that what you say is not as important as how you listen. By simply directing the conversation to the caller's emotional hungers, being a nonjudgmental sounding-board, the person will usually find her own answers. Be accepting and attentive; this is what you can hope someone will do for you.

Here are some of the responses we suggest when receiving an outreach call:

"I'm glad you called. Tell me what's going on in your life right now."

"What happened right before you started thinking about food or overeating?"

"What do you think you really need right now?"

"I'm glad you had the courage to call; it will inspire me to make a phone call myself the next time I want to hurt myself with food."

"This is hard to say because I really care about you, but it is not a good time for me to talk. I wonder if you could call someone else and call me back tomorrow."

The healing received from phone calls to safe people occurs on two levels. First, we benefit from picking up the phone and breaking our chronic pattern of isolation. We also benefit because we get to receive the attention we need from a loving, supportive person. Reaching out to safe people before, during, or after a binge is a direct route to feeding our emotional hungers.

Writing, drawing, or painting are other excellent paths for finding out about what is going on inside you. One idea is to simply take out paper and a pen and begin to write (or draw) when you have the need to eat, but sense you're not really hungry. You don't need to know what you're going to write about. Just write. And in this free-style writing exercise, don't worry about grammar, spelling, logic or legibility. Just put the pen to paper and let your thoughts and feelings roll! Write anything that you do know, and what you don't know will usually follow. This exercise is for your eyes alone. No one else needs to read it (though you could share it with a safe person). Safely expressing your feelings is the opposite of bingeing. You may not feel immediate relief, but don't give up. Once your heart and soul know there are safe places and safe people with whom you can be real, you will begin to feel better, and you will stop turning to food when you are emotionally hungry.

As you begin to stop overeating or undereating, you'll also begin to understand why you did so in the first place. These are usually one word reasons like: sadness, fear, anger or loneliness. When emotions are acknowledged and expressed in a safe and healthy manner, they become quite manageable and will pass by like leaves floating by on a stream. Overeating or undereating is an attempt to get your own attention, to give yourself something that you really need. So often, though, that need is intangible; it cannot be found in bags of cookies, containers of ice-cream, or in dietary restrictions. When you have learned (and you can learn this) to distinguish between your emotional and physical hunger, both types of hunger then become barometers to help you know what you need. This, we have found, is very different from experiencing hunger as a dreaded enemy.

It is okay to eat when you are hungry and to cry when you are sad. But ice cream will never alleviate sadness, and potato chips will not subdue anger. What is it you're hungry for right now?

❧ *Journey One*

*Date:*_____

1. a. List some times in the past week when you ate and were not physically hungry. Try to remember where you were, what you were doing, and what you were feeling. What happened to those feelings?

    _____

    _____

    _____

    _____

    _____

    _____

    _____

    b. Now list some times in the past week when you did not eat, even though you were physically hungry. What were your reasons for not eating?

    _____

    _____

    _____

    _____

    _____

    _____

    _____

2. What are some of the physical symptoms you experience when you are physically hungry?

    _____

    _____

    _____

    _____

    _____

    _____

3. How can you differentiate physical from emotional hunger if you are not sure?

_____

_____

_____

_____

_____

_____

4. How were you taught to confuse emotional and physical hungers? What rules or behaviors might your parents or others have passed on to you that resulted in your need to:

     a) eat in order to try to feel better?

     b) eat when you're not physically hungry?

     c) deprive yourself of food when you are physically hungry?

_____

_____

_____

_____

_____

_____

_____

_____

5.   a. Circle below all the emotions you are currently feeling.

Happy

Sad

Angry

Scared

Lonely

Ashamed

Peaceful

Hurt

Other:

b. Now imagine that each of the emotions you circled could speak. What would each say?

Examples:

Sad: "I'm so sad my best friend moved away."

Angry: "I'm furious that my family made fun of my weight when I was a child."

Hurt: "I've been living in your stomach for too long. I wish you would let me out."

---

c. Ask each of the above feelings what it truly needs right now and then write the responses below. (If it is too hard for you to imagine what you need, try instead to imagine your best friend or a small child expressing the above statements. What do you sense they might need?)

Examples:

Sad: "I need you to stop shoving food down my throat and let me cry."

Angry: "It was bad enough that everyone else picked on me. I need you to stop doing it now."

Hurt: "I need to be comforted. Could you please stop ignoring me and talk to a good friend? There are so many hurts. I need to have them heard."

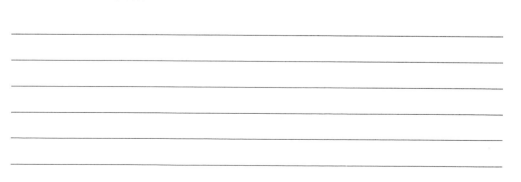

🌿 *Journey Two*

*Date:*_____

1.   a. List some times in the past week when you ate and were not physically hungry. Try to remember where you were, what you were doing, and what you were feeling. What happened to those feelings?

_____

_____

_____

_____

_____

_____

_____

_____

_____

_____

b. Now list some times in the past week when you did not eat, even though you were physically hungry. What were your reasons for not eating?

_____

_____

_____

_____

_____

_____

_____

_____

_____

_____

_____

_____

2. List possible ways to fill your emotional hungers (even if you are unable to do so at this time):

_____

_____

_____

_____

_____

_____

3. Circle items from the above list that you may be willing to try. What makes it difficult for you to try them? What would make it easier?

_____

_____

_____

_____

_____

_____

_____

_____

_____

4. What foods do you turn to for various feelings?

Examples: potato chips when angry
ice cream when lonely

_____

_____

_____

_____

_____

_____

❧ *Journey Three*

Date:_____

1. Reflect upon the last few times you ate. Were you physically hungry? How do you feel about your food choices and the manner in which you ate?

_____

_____

_____

_____

_____

_____

_____

_____

_____

_____

_____

2.   a. On a scale of 1-10 (1 being the least hungry, 10 being the most), how emotionally hungry are you right now?

1   5   10

_____

Not Hungry   Very Hungry

b. What are you emotionally hungry for right now?

_____

_____

_____

_____

_____

_____

_____

3. List some possible ways to fill your emotional hungers (even if you are unable to do so at this time):

_____

_____

_____

_____

_____

4. Circle items from the previous list that you are willing to try. Of the items left, what makes it difficult for you to try them?

_____

_____

_____

_____

_____

5. Who met your emotional needs when you were young? In what ways?

_____

_____

_____

_____

_____

_____

6. Looking back on Journeys One and Two, what do you notice about how you have or have not changed in relation to physical vs. emotional hungers?

_____

_____

_____

_____

_____

_____

_____

This sign designates what we will call a Spontaneous Road Trip. A Spontaneous Road Trip is akin to deciding to go off the beaten path and explore unknown territory. When you arrive at this sign in your workbook, we encourage you to do whatever you want on this page. You can use it to express anything going on for you at this time. You can draw, write spontaneously about your thoughts and feelings, make a collage, write a poem, insert a photograph of yourself... anything that will help you explore and record this current part of your Journey. (Remember there is no right or wrong way to do this!)

❦ *Journey Four*

*Date:*_____

1. Do some reflecting on the last few times you ate. Were you physically hungry? How do you feel about your food choices and the manner in which you ate?

_____

_____

_____

_____

_____

_____

2. What progress do you notice in your ability to distinguish physical from emotional hunger?

_____

_____

_____

_____

_____

_____

3. What are you currently emotionally hungry for?

_____

_____

_____

_____

_____

_____

4. What would it take to fill your current emotional hungers? Are you willing to do this? Why or why not?

_____

_____

_____

_____

_____

_____

_____

_____

5. Write about one time recently when you honored and filled an emotional hunger. What happened? What was it like?

_____

_____

_____

_____

_____

_____

_____

_____

_____

_____

6. What percentage of the time are you currently listening to and honoring your:

a. physical hunger?

_____

b. emotional hunger?

_____

Chapter 10

Diet vs. Live-It

The central concept behind this book is that in order to overcome problems with food and weight, we need to abandon the notion of "diets" and create a new way to live our lives. The word diet includes the word "die." It implies weakness, deprivation and starvation. Conversely, Live-It implies health, aliveness, and vitality. A diet is about restricting food. A Live-It is about having a sane, fulfilling relationship with food. Diets are about diminishing ourselves. Live-Its are about becoming ourselves more fully.

When we try to lose weight on a diet, we end up losing a lot more in the process; we lose our ability to concentrate, our ability to trust our bodies and our desires, our energy, our capacity to have intimate relationships, and we lose our awareness of the issues in our lives that may be problematic and in need of attention. We become singularly focused on food and weight. In a sense, we lose our lives, believing they'll begin again when we're thin. For most people, however, that day never comes.

Are diets working for you? We bet they're not. It may be time to take a good look at whether you want to continue turning to them for help with your food and weight problems. Below is a list of diet myths.

Myth #1
Someone else knows better than you what you should eat.

Every diet is based on the assumption that someone else knows better than you what your body needs and wants for energy, nutrition, and pleasure. Although it's important to understand good nutrition, nobody else, including world-renowned doctors, can possibly know when you are hungry and when you are not. You are the only one who can know if your hunger is emotional or physical. You are the only one who can feel the needs of your body at any particular moment. Having ignored your body's needs for so long, you may not know how to listen to it. To learn this, you will need support from people you know and trust, not formulas from strangers.

It is becoming common knowledge that diets do not work, so many diet companies are slashing the word "diet" from their marketing campaigns. Don't be fooled; a diet by any other name is still a diet. Whether they call it a "plan" or a "lifestyle change," if someone else is determining what foods you should put in your mouth, it's still a diet.

Myth #2
All you need to do is stick to a certain diet and you'll lose excess weight, then maintain your ideal weight.

The truth is, all diets end, but life continues. If you don't address the problems that cause your excessive eating, you will continue your old relationship with food when the diet ends. Most people who lose weight on diets eventually gain it back—with a rebate! Depriving your body of food damages your metabolism and eventually causes weight gain. A quick survey of your own history with diets, as well as of other people you know who have tried numerous diets, will show you that what you thought was a personal failure was not. Dieting contributes to weight gain.

Myth #3
You can control your weight and your eating by prohibiting yourself from eating certain foods.

Have you ever tried telling a child not to do something? What happened? Have you ever tried to tell yourself not to eat something? Did it work? The more forbidden an activity or a food is, the more desirable it becomes. The more we deprive ourselves of something, the more focused on it we become. Besides, food is not the problem. The way we cope with life is the problem. Prohibiting ourselves from eating a particular food does nothing to address our underlying emotions. What it does do is create feelings of rebelliousness and deprivation that lead to an obsessive desire for that food.

Myth #4
The way your body is now is unacceptable.

Many of us have unrealistic ideas of how our bodies should look. We base these ideas on images from the media. Actresses and models often starve themselves, vomit, or exercise viciously in order to create the bodies we see on television and in films and magazines. Magazine photos are often tampered with to make bodies appear flawless and thinner than they actually are.

Real people come in many shapes and sizes. All bodies are different. Trying to conform to one particular look is a losing battle. Your current body size may be a result of this battle. It is more appropriate to feel sadness and compassion for your body than it is to view it with disgust and self-hatred.

Myth #5
Changing your weight will solve your problems.

Losing weight may solve some problems. For example, weighing less may make you feel healthier, it may be easier to find clothes, and it may keep people from ridiculing you. But losing weight does not solve your food or body image issues. Nor does it solve the problems (like unresolved anger, grief, or pain) that caused you to turn to excess food or deprivation in the first place. These issues and their causes will continue to affect you even after you lose weight. This is why most people regain their weight after losing it on diets. You can be sure that if you don't address and heal the underlying issues that caused you to overeat, you will most certainly gain the weight back. (You still need it.) You cannot fix a serious engine problem in your car by giving the car a new paint job. A diet may give you the illusion of solving a problem, but it is just that, an illusion. The diet industry makes billions off of this mirage.

If diets don't work, what should you do about your food problems? We recommend that you develop a "Live-It" in place of a "Die-It." A Live-It encompasses the ways in which you live with and handle your eating, your emotions, your thinking and your spiritual hungers. A Live-It changes according to your stage of recovery, your body's needs, and your personal preferences.

A compulsive eater doesn't automatically stop overeating and suddenly find the ability to eat only when hungry. A bulimic doesn't go from bingeing and purging to calmly eating a sandwich and chips for lunch. And an anorexic is not going to go from a starvation diet to three nutritious meals a day. Each of these transitions will involve many steps and lots of support.

In the Transition and Early Stages of Recovery (see pg. 17) there are so many ingrained and mixed-up beliefs, along with unresolved hurts and emotions, that most of us are unable to hear or listen to our inner wisdom. During this time, people may need daily, or even meal-by-meal support in determining what to eat. While you may need to create more structure around your eating, doing so in the isolated ways you did when dieting is not going to work. You cannot focus solely on the food. Your relationships, your thinking, and your buried and unresolved emotions will all have to be dealt with. Rest assured that as you continue on this Journey, your food choices will become easier, and your eating more natural.

Imagine your Live-It as a four-legged stool. One leg of the stool represents your physical needs. The next leg of the stool represents your emotional needs. The third leg stands for your intellectual needs, and the fourth leg represents your spiritual needs. In order for the stool (your Live-It) to remain standing, sturdy, and upright, all four legs need to be strong. In other words, in order for you to stop your compulsive behaviors with food, your physical, emotional, intellectual, and spiritual needs must all be attended to.

People who focus only on the physical aspects of a Live-It (i.e. food and exercise) and do not address the emotional, intellectual, and spiritual aspects, never seem to end their weight battles. Those who seek therapy for their emotions, without daily support for their self-destructive thinking and eating patterns, also seem to stay stuck. People who focus only on an intellectual understanding of food and weight problems never obtain the spiritual and emotional growth necessary for a full recovery. Those attending only to spiritual aspects of a Live-It continue to eat over their unresolved emotions. But people who focus on, and get support in, all four areas eventually make it through the Transition Stage into Early Recovery and, eventually, Ongoing Recovery. This is the stage when you are really able to hear and respond to your inner voice, when you actually move beyond your body obsession, to finally make peace with food.

Remembering that a Live-It is ever-changing, depending on where you are at any given point in your recovery, we will now describe some general philosophies and benefits of a Live-It.

Principle #1
You decide what to eat.

A Live-It is yours and no one else's. Only you know what is best for your body. Only you know what foods you like and dislike and what amounts are right for you at any given time. This may change from day to day, and you are the only one who can monitor the changes.

Some people need structure, and some need to let go of structure. Some people need to avoid certain binge foods, others need to stop restricting themselves. If you cannot yet trust yourself, we encourage you to find healthy, supportive people to help you make sure you are not depriving or being dishonest with yourself. You might find such a person in a support group.

Here are some of the different ways our clients define their Live-Its:

a. "I eat 3 meals a day, anything I want, except my 4 personal binge foods."

b. "My Live-It is guilt-free eating. I either let go of the guilt, let go of the food, or I eat the food and get immediate help with the guilt."

c. "Every time I think of food, I get quiet and ask my heart if I am truly physically hungry. If I am, I eat. If I'm not, I find out what I really need."

d. "No bingeing, no dieting, no purging."

e. "Healthy eating 85% of the time. Sane eating 100%."

f. "I eat what nourishes me in ways that nurture me."

g. "I treat myself kindly in all ways, and when I am unable to do so, I seek out support."

h. "I try to follow my heart at all times and give or get for myself whatever I am physically, emotionally or spiritually hungry for."

Principle #2
All foods are acceptable, in moderation.

Many of us have tried to eliminate specific foods attributing them to our problems with weight. If this were so, few of us would still have food and weight problems. We would have solved the problems by simply eliminating the foods. Granted, there can be health reasons for avoiding certain foods, but it is important to make a distinction between our food, weight, and body image issues and valid medical reasons for specific diets. For example, being allergic to dairy products is a good reason not to eat cheese. However, avoiding cheese because you fear it and think it will make you fat, only supports your obsession with food and weight—and that keeps you unhealthy.

So, rather than telling yourself unhelpful statements like this food is "good" or "bad," "fattening" or "fat-free," try asking yourself, "Would a person who is sane, moderate and self-loving eat this right now?" If the answer is "yes" we encourage you to trust yourself and allow yourself to eat. If you are not sure, we recommend that you reach out to a safe person for support in getting clear. If the answer is "no" we hope you will attend to the emotional needs that are indicated by your craving.

During the Early Recovery Stage, there will be times when you'll know that eating your favorite snack food is likely to trigger a binge. Using Loving Limits to avoid that food until you can handle it makes sense. For example, if you are full of unresolved feelings and you know that eating a few chocolate raisins will lead you to devouring the entire bag, it may be a more loving choice to hold off from eating any until you can get emotional support. Once your emotional needs are met, chocolate raisins will become safe to eat again (if you even still want them).

Principle #3
A Live-It is not just about food.

Most diets are one-size-fits-all food plans. While a Live-It does involve the subject of food, it also includes much more. A Live-It requires that you develop compassion and self-love. A Live-It challenges you to live with integrity and to deepen your level of honesty. It calls for you to improve your ability to relate to and connect with others. It involves understanding your past hurts and moving toward healing and forgiveness. It requires learning how to be present and not abandoning yourself, even in difficult or scary situations. And when it comes to food, it's not restriction that's important, but being profoundly honest about what, how, and why you are eating.

Principle #4
There is nothing wrong with you, and you do not need to punish yourself by dieting.

You may have food problems, you may weigh more than you like, you may have body image problems, but you are not bad! You are not weak, you are not lazy, you do not need willpower. You have challenges and you have struggles. You have unresolved inner pain. You do not need to be punished. In fact, punishment only makes you feel worse. If punishment was effective, you probably wouldn't be reading this book right now.

Principle #5
Reaching out to supportive and understanding people is vital to a successful Live-It.

When you're dealing with food and body issues you need compassion and understanding. If you have problems with food, you are having a problem with life. You are having feelings you need to deal with. You also need to connect with a safe person and with "the part of you that knows." Going on a diet or planning future deprivation does not help you. Calling someone who is supportive and understanding does. Speaking to yourself compassionately and lovingly does.

Principle #6
A Live-It enables you to make gradual and long-lasting changes.

If you have a problem with your weight, you need to address your problem, not your weight. There are important reasons why you struggle or are obsessed with food, weight, and body image. The changes you need to make must first take place on the inside; the outside will follow later (if necessary). Your heart and soul and feelings need to heal before your body can reflect your inner transformation. With a Live-It, any weight loss or gain will be slow and gradual. Your weight may fluctuate as you encounter roadblocks on your Journey. As you work through and heal these inner problem areas, you will find that the changes occurring on the inside and the outside are profound and permanent.

Principle #7
A Live-It never ends.

A Live-It will evolve and change as you do, but it will continue for as long as you live. There's no "blowing it," going off it or starting "tomorrow." If you have a problem with food, you view it as an indicator that you are having a problem with something in your life. Instead of trying to control your food, you focus on what may be bothering you. You seek out supportive people with whom you can honestly communicate, and you identify and resolve the feelings that are causing you to turn to food. Your Live-It may change according to your needs and where you are on your Journey. If your Live-It becomes unworkable or unhealthy, you reevaluate and alter it.

Following is Andrea's story about her Live-It:

> *The best thing about my Live-It is that it's mine. And it's a Live-It I can live with. There's nothing to break or start over. I follow my heart and my hunger, not some plan written by some doctor or determined by some set of rules. I think it is important to convey that my Live-It has evolved over time and still changes according to my stage of recovery, my needs, and my lifestyle.*
>
> *When I first began my Journey, I needed some structure. I made it as simple as three meals a day and no purging. I had so many unresolved and unexpressed emotions, I couldn't trust myself to know when I was physically or emotionally hungry. I felt empty inside, and I had spent years trying to fill my emptiness with food. I did not know how to eat sanely and moderately. It was very easy for me to inadvertently slip into bingeing. I also had to watch out for my tendency to deprive myself of food. I came to understand that undereating was dangerous for me and was usually followed by a binge. Because I was not able to trust myself with food, I needed a lot of help and support from people who were on the same Journey. (Those who weren't, though they had good intentions, often gave me inappropriate advice.)*
>
> *I began to let go of the concept of "good" and "bad" foods by distinguishing between foods I thought I "shouldn't" eat and foods that were difficult for me because they were likely to set off a binge. I needed to have some Loving Limits without becoming too rigid. This often felt like a very thin line and was not something I could figure out by myself (if I could have, I wouldn't have developed an eating disorder in the first place!)*

With help from my support people (my therapist and members of the recovery groups I attended), I made a decision to do my best to refrain from my personal binge foods. The structure of "three meals a day with nothing in between" helped me tremendously in defining a beginning and an end to my eating and by reassuring me that I deserved and would be eating regular meals.

When I couldn't figure out what to eat at these meals, I would often imagine handing a beautiful tray of food to someone I love. I'd picture a red rose in a silver vase, a cloth napkin, a pot of tea, a china plate and fine silverware. Then I'd let my imagination come up with a lovely balanced meal to go on the plate. And that's how I would decide what to feed myself.

As I said, I needed a lot of support. So I made a lot of phone calls. I used my support system to help me figure out whether I was physically or emotionally hungry, what the best food choices were for me, and whether or not I was setting myself up for a binge by depriving myself or by eating foods that felt unsafe. The calls got easier to make over time. I called people who were on the same path, but ahead of me, knowing that they would understand my needs.

After some time, I began to trust myself more around food. I didn't need to call people quite so frequently. Increasingly, I knew exactly what I was feeling, what I hungered for, and what I needed. I still made (and make) phone calls, but out of a loving choice rather than out of desperation. As a result of the emotional work I was doing, I began to feel less empty. I did not crave food to fill me as often. I began to know when I was physically hungry and was able to incorporate snacking into my Live-It. Although there were many days when I still overate, they became fewer over time. And when I did overeat, my bingeing didn't go on for as long as it had in the past.

Today, my Live-It is not only about food. I have made a peace treaty with myself and with my body. My Live-It is about treating myself lovingly in all aspects of my life. When it comes to hunger, if I am emotionally hungry I know that no food will satisfy me, and instead I seek emotional and spiritual ways to fill those hungers. If I am physically hungry, I feed myself whatever my body wants, be it carrots or carrot cake.

We know that a Live-It is not as clear-cut as a diet, and that it involves more emotional, mental, social, and spiritual changes. We also know that Live-Its are more successful than diets, easier than diets, gentler than diets, healthier than diets (and cheaper, too!). It's worth going through all the changes and learning how to permanently live with food rather than without it.

🌿 *Journey One*

*Date:*_____

1. What foods do you blame for your food and weight problems?

_____

_____

_____

_____

2. What do you think happens when you eat these foods?

_____

_____

_____

_____

_____

_____

3. At this point, what would you consider "perfect eating?"

_____

_____

_____

_____

_____

_____

4. How realistic is "perfect eating" in terms of your ability to stick to it and maintain health?

_____

_____

_____

_____

5. On a scale of 1 to 10, (1 being extreme rigidity, 10 being complete flexibility), how would you rate your just-described eating plan?

_____

6. Using the same scale, how would you describe a "5" eating plan?

_____
_____
_____
_____
_____
_____

7. Would it be appropriate to have this number "5" plan be your Live-It? Why, or why not?

_____
_____
_____
_____
_____
_____

8. Looking back to some of the Live-It examples on page 149, how might you currently define your Live-It? How would it be different from a diet?

_____
_____
_____
_____
_____
_____
_____
_____

✖ *Journey Two*

*Date:*_____

1	5	10
Bingeing	Live-It	Dieting
(overeating)	(moderate eating)	(undereating)

1. Mark on the above scale where you are today.

2. What feelings do you associate with the different parts of the scale?

1	5	10
Bingeing	Live-It	Dieting

3. What fears keep you from being more relaxed about your food and weight?

_____

_____

_____

_____

_____

4. If you were to define your Live-It just for today what would it be?

_____

_____

_____

_____

_____

5. a. Write a letter to your eating disorder, as if it's your friend:

Dear Eating Disorder,

_____

_____

_____

_____

_____

_____

_____

_____

_____

_____

b. Write a letter to your eating disorder, as if it's your enemy:

Dear Eating Disorder,

_____

_____

_____

_____

_____

_____

_____

_____

_____

_____

_____

❧ *Journey Three*

*Date:*_____

1	5	10
Bingeing	Live-It	Dieting
(overeating)	(moderate eating)	(undereating)

1. Mark on the above scale where you are today.

2. What feelings lead you to bingeing?

_____

_____

_____

_____

_____

_____

3. What feelings lead you to dieting?

_____

_____

_____

_____

4. What have you learned about the effects of bingeing, and/or dieting, on your feelings?

_____

_____

_____

_____

_____

_____

5. Write a good-bye letter to dieting. If you're not ready to say good-bye, write why you're not.

Dear Dieting,

_____

_____

_____

_____

_____

_____

_____

6. What is your idea of a Live-It today? How is this different from your ideas about it in Journey One?

_____

_____

_____

_____

_____

_____

_____

1	5	10
Never listening to body cues (bingeing & dieting)		Always listening to body cues (healthy eating)

7.   a. On the above scale, where were you when you started this book? Where are you now?

b. What would it take for you to move further to the right on the scale?

_____

_____

_____

_____

🌿 *Journey Four*

*Date:*_____

1. List below all the thoughts and behaviors that you now consider to be diet mentality.

_____

_____

_____

_____

_____

_____

2. Looking at the myths that begin on page 146, which do you still believe?

_____

_____

_____

3. Describe your current Live-It.

_____

_____

_____

_____

_____

_____

4. Look back at Journey Three, Question #7. Mark where you are on that scale now. What would it take for you to move a little further to the right on that scale?

_____

_____

_____

_____

This sign designates what we will call a Spontaneous Road Trip. A Spontaneous Road Trip is akin to deciding to go off the beaten path and explore unknown territory. When you arrive at this sign in your workbook, we encourage you to do whatever you want on this page. You can use it to express anything going on for you at this time. You can draw, write spontaneously about your thoughts and feelings, make a collage, write a poem, insert a photograph of yourself... anything that will help you explore and record this current part of your Journey. (Remember there is no right or wrong way to do this!)

Chapter 11

Weight Control vs. Natural Weight

"But if I don't control my weight, I'll blow up like a balloon!"
"I worked so hard to lose the weight, and now I'm gaining it all back!"
"I know the kind of foods I should be eating. I just don't
understand why I can't eat that way!"

Many of our clients live in constant fear and distrust of their bodies. They tend to think of their bodies as separate and dangerous entities, like wild animals that need to be caged and tamed. After all the deprivation, neglect, and stuffed emotions, it's not surprising that your body feels ravenous and out of control. Starving for nutrients and nurturing, it seems to have a will of its own. It is important to understand, however, that this disassociation from your body is the result of how you have treated yourself. It is not your body's natural state.

When children grow up in homes with ample and healthy food, loving attention, and understanding, they eat when they're hungry and refuse to eat when they're not. Their bodies are naturally wise about what they do and do not need. With this wisdom, children's bodies grow at their uniquely perfect pace. Without any external control, bodies develop a particular shape; weight alternately increases and stabilizes and continues to do so throughout the process of puberty and maturation.

Why, then, do we come to believe we need to take control of this natural process? First of all, we live in a culture that has idealized thinness, and tragically rendered "fat" a dirty word. Naturally we assumed that getting thin would solve our problems and make us feel lovable. Secondly, we may have felt hopeless and out of control in our families or in a traumatic situation and found we could gain some semblance of control by losing weight, a painstaking effort that also served to distract us from our original problems. Finally, the desire to manipulate our bodies may have begun when we were young and discovered something about our bodies that we did not like (or that someone else did not like).

Many of our clients can recall a specific moment when they began to hate parts (or all) of their bodies. They also have a clear recollection of the first time someone else shamed or violated parts (or all) of their bodies. Rather than challenge such criticism (which may have had some or no basis in reality), many of us think we need to, instead, change ourselves in order to meet the expectations of others or to look like (or be like) someone else. Out of our natural desire to be loved and accepted, we spend many years of our lives trying to change our bodies into something they were not intended to be. Unfortunately, if we are unable to feel positive about who we are, changing the way our body looks won't help us to do so. Additionally, manipulating our body size and shape takes so much time and effort, we end up with little energy left for living life, developing our strengths and talents, or working on the real problems underlying our food dilemmas: low self-esteem and lack of relationship skills. After all, if we had grown up in an esteeming environment, we would have realized that it's okay to have a body that is different from others' and that everyone's body is unique and special — including ours! If we had been taught relationship skills when we were young, we would have known how to tell people when their criticism hurt us, and we could have asked them to stop. Instead, many of us spend the rest of our lives trying to change ourselves.

As therapists and as women who have battled with weight issues, we have found that most people who work hard at controlling their bodies never actually get to a point where they feel satisfied with their weight. What a frustrating and painful way to live! The healthy alternative to constantly trying to control the shape of your body is to befriend and listen to it, and give it what it needs. Doing so will lead you to your *Natural Weight*, the weight that your body settles into when you eat according to your body's real needs. Finding your natural weight is a process that takes time. This process challenges years of familial and cultural beliefs that have taught you not to listen to your body. It also challenges the idea that you are not lovable and can somehow become lovable by losing weight.

Finding your natural weight involves gradually trusting your body and trusting food. Trusting your body means trusting your emotional feelings and needs, as well as your physical feelings and needs. Trusting food involves letting go of the rules and fears you have about certain foods.

Many of us have numerous strict rules when it comes to food. "Salad is good." "Dessert is bad." "Don't eat fats." On and on. Have you ever experienced the craziness of overeating "good" foods in order to avoid a "forbidden food" only to end up eating large quantities of both? After years of living by rigid rules, when we first let go of control we often find ourselves gravitating toward the very foods we feared most. Don't panic. When your body and soul know, beyond a shadow of a doubt, that they absolutely can have these foods, you will stop craving them so intensely. However, at first you may not be able to eat such foods with freedom. Getting to the point of freedom with food is a process. It involves traveling many of the recovery roads you're exploring in this workbook (e.g. reaching out, acknowledging feelings, Loving Limits, Rainbow Thinking, etc.).

The following is Marsea's experience of how developing a sense of freedom with a particular food was part of her process in attaining her natural weight.

Before my recovery, I was obsessed with chocolate chip cookies. I sometimes spent entire days driving to different places in my search of the perfect cookie (you know, the one that would satisfy you forever!). I sometimes spent entire evenings mixing up batter, only to devour it all before it even got into the oven. Of course, I considered cookies to be "bad" foods, and on my "good" days I never ate them. I thought that as fat as I was, I shouldn't eat cookies if I truly wanted to lose weight like I said I did.

When I started my recovery, I couldn't have cookies in my Live-It because I was so fearful of them. My panic about eating even one would drive me to eat too many. Also, because I still considered cookies "bad," the part of me that liked them always thought, "This is the last time I will ever eat chocolate chip cookies," and, therefore, I wanted to eat as many as I possibly could. After all, I'd never get the chance to eat them again!

Eventually, because I could never seem to cut cookies out of my life, I began to realize that it didn't kill me to eat them. In fact, the more I allowed them to be part of my Live-It, the less fear they instilled, and the less desperate I was to have them. My process of letting go of my fear and judgment about cookies, along with numerous calls I made for support, and working on the emotional issues that caused me to numb myself out with cookies in the first place, led me to freedom from my cookie obsession. I am no longer controlled by cookies. If I notice them becoming problematic, I turn to my support system until I can figure out what feelings I am trying to suppress. When I handle my feelings, cookies are no longer an issue.

Today, a cookie is just a cookie. I can eat one, or not eat one. I can even love cookies at times — because they're not an obsession. Ironically, when cookies were a "bad" food, and I was trying to avoid them in order to control my weight, I weighed a lot more than I do today. Decriminalizing cookies (and other "bad" foods), and letting go of weight "control" were important aspects to the eventual attainment of my natural weight.

Many of us have been living by rule books, and trying to manipulate our weight for so long that we have no idea what our natural weight is. Often we have an irrational fear that our body would just keep growing and growing if we didn't control it. But, unless you have a medical condition that causes weight gain, this is only true if you are not addressing your emotional needs.

Also, many people have a distorted body image. We believe that we have gained weight, when in fact we haven't. We believe that we're fat when, in fact, we aren't. This is because we connect feelings with "fat" and can't tell the difference. We know we feel something, but since we can't identify the feeling, we think it must be about weight. "Huge feelings" can make us feel huge!

If you feel out of control regarding your weight, and a doctor has ruled out any medical problems, the only solution is to focus on your inner needs. Weight control is not a solution. In fact, weight control leads to "weight out-of-control."

A person's natural weight can be affected by numerous factors, including: genetics, metabolism, age, health, food preferences, activity level, menstrual cycle, stress, and damage accrued by years of dieting. Some of these factors can cause your weight to fluctuate. This is normal. Such fluctuations mean that your natural weight is not one single number — it's a range.

When we are controlling our weight, we often experience much greater fluctuations — first losing many pounds, then gaining them back, plus more. This causes us to become fearful of *any* change; we panic if we see the scale going up even one pound. For this reason, it is often helpful to put away the scale once we begin trusting our body to find its natural weight. Later on this Journey, you may find that using the scale occasionally can be helpful, but only if you use it as a "reality check," rather than a "self-worth check." The difference between the two is whether or not you can be objective. A reality check is weighing yourself just to satisfy your curiosity. A self-worth check is weighing yourself to determine if you're presentable or lovable or successful enough, or to see if you should be allowed to eat that day. If you think that seeing a number on the scale could cause you to overeat, undereat, obsess, or feel badly about yourself, we recommend that you not use it. Weighing yourself is a choice, not a necessity.

Marsea:

Whenever I was on my latest weight loss scheme, I weighed myself many times a day — when I woke up, after going to the bathroom or showering, after eating, after exercising, etc.

When I began losing weight on my Journey of Recovery, I was tempted to start in on my old weighing routines. Yet I found that often when I weighed myself, I would lose my peaceful relationship with food and begin eating compulsively again. If I had lost weight, I saw it as reason to eat extra food. If I had gained weight, I felt hopeless and used food to numb out; then, I'd vow to eat less at my next meal, which only caused me to feel deprived and panicked, which led me to eat more. If my weight had stayed the same, I'd be totally frustrated and would, of course, "need" food to mellow out.

I realized that weighing was dangerous for me, so I got rid of my scale. After awhile I'd get really curious about my weight, and feel it was too extreme to never know what I weighed, so I decided to weigh myself once every other month at a local medical center. I knew, though, that weighing was still a tricky situation, so when the time came, I asked a friend, who was a very safe person, if she would accompany me. She actually felt the same need for support around weighing that I did. On our way to the center we talked about our fears, expectations, and issues around our weight. Upon arrival, we weighed ourselves, then we left and sat outside under some trees. There we shared our feelings about what the scale said, and we made plans for getting through the rest of the day without using food.

We went on several "weight dates." They were very powerful, and healing. We took weighing out of the private realm. No longer were we alone with the scale and our anxiety. We were able to break our unhealthy patterns around weighing. We got the support we needed so we could handle our feelings about our weight without using food to cope with those feelings.

Today, I am at my natural weight, which is 60-70 lbs. less than what it was then. And I can look at my weight on the scale, without turning to food. Letting go of my attempts to control my weight by monitoring it, and getting support with my feelings about my weight were two of the elements that helped me find serenity and attain my natural weight.

When you eat according to your body's real needs, for an ongoing period of time, your body automatically finds its natural weight. *Your* natural weight, not anyone else's. Once at your natural weight, you may discover that you actually like your body at that weight. What a relief! On the other hand, you may have difficulty accepting your natural body weight. You may need to grieve the loss of your "fantasy body" before coming to peace with the unique body that is actually yours. Although experiencing grief can be a challenging part of this Journey, it is often followed by an immense amount of relief. Allowing yourself to experience your feelings of anger, sadness, and frustration about never being able to have the "perfect" body paves the road toward accepting your natural weight. The peace then comes from accepting yourself as a real person — as opposed to an incomplete person struggling to become "ideal."

Of course, accepting yourself is not necessarily an easy or automatic task. Here are some of the things we did to help us achieve body acceptance at different points along our Journeys.

Transition Stage:
-Listen to tapes about body acceptance (see Appendix D).
-Read books on body acceptance (see Appendix D).
-Repeat affirmations such as "I love my body," "My body deserves love," "I am acceptable as I am."
-Address body hatred in group and/or individual therapy.

Early Recovery:
-Address emotions, such as grief, hurt, or rage, so that body obsession isn't needed as a distraction from these feelings.
-When you beome aware of body hatred, complete the sentence: If I wasn't distracted by body hatred right now, I would thinking about or feeling . . .
-Seek out beautiful, full-bodied women as role models. (Check out *Mode Magazine!*)

Ongoing Recovery:
-Look in the mirror and try to:
    1. Show compassion for how your body got the way it is.
    2. Appreciate what you do have and what your body does do for you.
    3. Apologize to your body for hating it.
    4. Say, "I love you," or "I am trying to love you."

-Go places, such as spas, where nudity is acceptable, and practice being nude until it feels comfortable.

-Have someone who loves you (or do this yourself) touch, and love your most uncomfortable body parts.

We know that when you do any of these things, you will experience many feelings. (Even thinking of them probably has you terrified!) It is very important that you "bookend" these activities with support — call a safe person before and after. Writing about your feelings is also helpful.

Everybody has a different process with body acceptance. Here are some examples from our clients:

Tina, discovered that when she stopped dieting, found her Live-It and began to deal with her emotional pain, her weight began to slowly and naturally decrease. She said she was "losing pains" instead of pounds. She knew that as long as she continued to attend to her emotional needs, she would attain her natural weight. She didn't know what that weight would be, but she was ready to accept whatever it was.

Claire, however, found that no matter how much she healed from her inner pain, her weight remained the same. She was glad she wasn't gaining, but frustrated that she wasn't losing. She knew that reverting back to dieting and food control would only make her more obsessed and unhappy, so she began the painful, yet profoundly worthwhile, process of making peace with her body. She was no longer willing to spend the rest of her life fighting a losing battle to try to make her body size smaller than it was meant to be. Today, Claire is a large, healthy woman who is relieved of her compulsive eating and weight obsession.

Another client, Felice, came to realize that her desired weight was unrealistic and unhealthy for her body; that, in fact, she needed to gain, not lose, weight in order to be at her natural size. Felice had spent many years undereating and abusing laxatives. When she began to eat regularly and abstain from laxatives she gained some weight. She was terrified that she would never stop gaining. But she stayed in close contact with other recovering people who also had to gain weight, and they gave her constant reassurance. One recovered laxative abuser told her to expect some swelling from water retention as her body adjusted to the absence of laxatives. Eventually, Felice's weight stabilized. Today she feels strong and healthy, and is relieved of her food and weight obsession.

If you are eating to suppress your feelings, you are probably not at your natural body weight. Nor are you weighing what nature intended your body to weigh if you are restricting your food intake or alternating between overeating and depriving yourself. It's important to remember, however, that finding your natural weight is not just about what you eat. It's about all the Journeys in this book. It's about how you live.

This sign designates what we will call a Spontaneous Road Trip. A Spontaneous Road Trip is akin to deciding to go off the beaten path and explore unknown territory. When you arrive at this sign in your workbook, we encourage you to do whatever you want on this page. You can use it to express anything going on for you at this time. You can draw, write spontaneously about your thoughts and feelings, make a collage, write a poem, insert a photograph of yourself... anything that will help you explore and record this current part of your Journey. (Remember there is no right or wrong way to do this!)

Journey One

*Date:*_____

1.   a. Write about your earliest memories of not liking your body or of someone criticizing or violating your body.

_____

_____

_____

_____

_____

     b. What do you want to say to the person who criticized or violated you?

_____

_____

_____

_____

_____

     c. What do you want to say to the part of you that got criticized or violated?

_____

_____

_____

_____

_____

     d. What do you want to say right now to your body?

_____

_____

_____

_____

_____

2. Where do you now get negative messages about your body size?

_____

_____

_____

_____

_____

3. Do you think you are currently at your natural weight ? Why or why not?

_____

_____

_____

_____

_____

_____

4. What do you do to try to control your weight? Does it work? How does it affect your life?

_____

_____

_____

_____

_____

5. What is your current relationship with the scale? How often do you weigh yourself? When you get off the scale, what do you tell yourself if you have gained/lost weight?

_____

_____

_____

_____

_____

6. How often did your mother weigh herself?

_____

7. Complete the following sentences:

a. Three rules I have in my food "rule book" are:

_____
_____
_____
_____
_____

b. Looking back on my ability to follow those rules, I see:

_____
_____
_____
_____
_____
_____

c. I'm afraid that if I gave up control of my weight then:

_____
_____
_____
_____
_____
_____
_____
_____
_____

❧ *Journey Two*

*Date:*_____

1. When and why did you first start trying to control your weight?

_____

_____

_____

_____

_____

2. What percentage of your time is spent each day on trying to control your weight? (Consider your thoughts as well as behaviors.)

_____

3. What do you do to try and control your weight? Does it work? How does it affect your life?

_____

_____

_____

_____

_____

_____

4. Do you think you are currently at your natural weight? If not, what keeps you from being at your natural weight? If you are, how does it feel? Are you at peace with it?

_____

_____

_____

_____

_____

5. Imagine what it would be like to no longer battle with your weight. Write below a description of whatever thoughts, images or feelings come to mind:

_____

_____

_____

_____

_____

_____

_____

_____

_____

_____

6. If your weight could speak right now, what would it say?

_____

_____

_____

_____

_____

_____

_____

_____

7. How would your Loving Voice respond?

_____

_____

_____

_____

_____

_____

_____

_____

❧ *Journey Three*

*Date:*_____

1. What percentage of your time is spent each day trying to control your weight? (Consider your thoughts as well as behaviors.) How does this compare to Journey Two?

_____

_____

_____

_____

_____

_____

2. How would you know if you were at your natural weight?

_____

_____

_____

_____

3. Do you think you are currently at your natural weight? If not, what keeps you from being there? If you are, how does it feel? Are you at peace with it?

_____

_____

_____

_____

_____

_____

_____

4. Use the space below to express any grief, anger or disappointment you are experiencing about not having your fantasy body. You can write, draw, write a poem, make a collage, or anything else that comes to mind.

5. How do you plan to respond to negative messages about your food or your weight? Give examples.

For example: If my mother comments on my food choices at dinner, I will say, "Mom, I really don't like it when you comment on what I eat. Please don't do it anymore."

If my father makes a snide comment about my weight, I will say, "I'm not sure what your intention is, but what you are saying is hurtful to me."

_____

_____

_____

_____

_____

_____

✵ *Journey Four*

*Date:*_____

1. What percentage of your time is spent each day trying to control your weight? (Consider your thoughts as well as behaviors.) How does this compare to Journey Three, Question #1?

_____

_____

_____

_____

2. Do you think you are at your natural weight? Why or why not?

_____

_____

_____

_____

_____

3. Are you willing to let your body adjust to its natural weight? Why or why not?

_____

_____

_____

_____

4. What do you think will happen if you continue to try to control your weight?

_____

_____

_____

_____

_____

5. What do you think will happen if you let go of trying to control your weight?

_____

_____

_____

_____

_____

6. How is your life different when you are not focusing on your weight?

_____

_____

_____

_____

_____

_____

7. What are some of the feelings/situations that trigger you to obsess about your weight?

_____

_____

_____

_____

_____

_____

8. List some alternative things you could do when you find yourself distracted by your weight.

_____

_____

_____

_____

_____

Chapter 12

Competition vs. Camaraderie

"At least I'm not the fattest one in the room."
"She's so good for ordering a salad."
"He's not doing the diet as well as I am."
"Look how fast she is on the treadmill."

These competitive thoughts make it appear as if we are in some invisible race to achieve the "perfect body," and our very lives depend on it. Many of us believe that somehow, if we just get thin enough, our feelings, our hearts and souls, our lives will be magically transformed. We become convinced that if we lose the weight that seems to be at the core of all our problems, we'll cross the finish line and will finally feel loved and connected to others in the ways we so deeply hunger for.

Competition for the "perfect body" is perpetuated by the media, which glorifies a far too narrow range of acceptable body types. In actuality, all bodies are different and unique. The unrealistic pursuit of model-like thinness causes us to constantly compete with each other in a race that goes nowhere. Many women feel threatened by thinner women, and many men feel threatened by more "buffed" men, rather than recognizing that we are all different, that there's room for all of us, and that we are much more than the shape of our bodies. In the race to be thin, everyone is the loser. The "winner" is left without genuine friendship, and the "less than best" person is filled with feelings of inadequacy. After all, how can people feel close to people who are judging them or liking them based on the shape of their bodies?

Competition takes many subtle forms. It can be heard in the conversations women have with each other; it can be seen in the jealous glance one woman gives another; it can be felt in the punishing ways we treat our bodies.

Many of our clients report that much of their conversation with other women consists of what we call *Fat Chat*. That is, complaining about eating or weight, gossip about who has gained or lost weight, conversations about the latest diets, discussions about cosmetic surgery procedures, etc. When we engage in Fat Chat, though we may feel momentarily bonded with the group, we are missing opportunities for more meaningful conversations about our lives and encouraging self-destructive and hurtful behaviors. By focusing on body and food concerns, we fail to converse about our feelings, our inner conflicts, our goals, our aspirations. In many circles, Fat Chat seems more acceptable.

Unfortunately, as early as preadolescence, we are encouraged to compare ourselves to others according to our appearance. We then tend to compete with our friends and put ourselves down, rather than maintain true friends and allies. When we are driven to compare ourselves with others, it is because we are in some way dissatisfied with who we are. Comparing ourselves to others is a sign of low self-esteem. When we feel okay about ourselves, we don't spend our time making comparisons — we just live. When we compare ourselves to others we usually end up feeling either superior or inferior. In either case, comparisons separate us, creating loneliness, isolation, alienation and, oftentimes, jealousy. These feelings contaminate, or even destroy, relationships.

The issue of jealousy, and what can happen when you address the underlying low self-esteem, is exemplified by Andrea's story about the beginning of her relationship with her husband:

> *Occasionally I'd have pangs of jealousy if I noticed Michael looking at another woman. My friends would tell me that it's perfectly normal for men to look at other women. They would make the point that, like paintings and beautiful flowers, people are simply interesting and enjoyable to look at. That helped my thinking, but it didn't change my feelings. I tried to tolerate it if I saw Michael turn his head, but silently I was comparing myself to the woman he was looking at. I'd think about which of us had better hair, nicer clothes, or who was thinner. Usually I'd end up making a sarcastic comment to Michael, and of course that pushed him away, when what I really needed was reassurance that he loved me.*
>
> *Finally I started to see that it was my job to turn my attitude around, not my partner's. My jealousy had more to do with my negative views about myself than with Michael's actions. (Of course, that would not be the case if, in my heart, I knew he was inappropriately flirting or being disrespectful to me.) No one else could change how I was feeling about myself. No one else could fix the part of me that felt pain. I began to understand this and to take responsibility for getting my inner needs met, particularly addressing the part of me that felt completely unlovable.*
>
> *A turning point came one day when we walked past a woman, and I noticed Michael noticing her. I silently talked to the part of me inside that was like a hurt little girl. I said to myself: "I know you felt hurt when Michael looked at that other woman. You are good enough, and you are special enough. You are beautiful, too." When Michael looked at me a few minutes later, he found an intact adult woman, rather than a hurt, blaming little girl. This*

shift in my inner dialogue, or "self talk," was a major turning point for me. Now that I can understand that jealousy and competition signal my need for love and reassurance, I can take responsibility for finding healthy ways to meet those needs. As a result, I have a more loving relationship with my husband, as well as with other women.

How we talk to ourselves (critical self-talk), and how we talk to others (Fat Chat), are two ways we perpetuate unhealthy competition. How we treat our bodies is another. Look inside any health club and you will see people trying to reshape their bodies so they can qualify for this perpetual race to fit in. Of course, there's nothing wrong with exercise, wanting to feel good physically, or valuing health and fitness. However, we have never seen weight loss or a muscular build bring peace to a hurt soul, or heal a history of emotional pain.

Though people who exercise are often admired and envied, exercise can become "too much of a good thing." Extreme exercise can be another form of bulimia. When it is used to counter binges, or as an expression of self-hatred, exercise becomes a form of purging and self-destruction. It can also be used as a distraction from problems that need to be addressed. Exercise has a place in a balanced life, but we'll never be satisfied with how our bodies look and feel until we deal with who we are on the inside and make peace with ourselves. When we push to sculpt our bodies while neglecting to develop our sense of self-love and inner worth, we end up unbalanced and dissatisfied. If we do not like ourselves to begin with, no matter how much we work on our physical bodies, we will never value who we are. In such instances, our motivation for exercise comes from a place of self-hatred and fear, and even a "perfect" body cannot eradicate those feelings.

When you compete in the race to be thin, your body usually pays a price. You may push yourself when you are exhausted, discount physical pain, or deprive yourself of nutrition. When you don't listen to and take care of your body, you increase your likelihood of injuries or illness.

Mistreating our bodies in order to gain the competitive edge is also seen in our obsession with fashion. How often have you stuffed yourself into clothes that were too tight? Worn uncomfortable but stylish shoes? Bought something you really couldn't afford but just had to have? Keeping up with perceived competitors in the "Who's-the-most-fashionable?" game can be an endless, unfulfilling cycle. The initial "high" of the new dress quickly leads to a "crash" when the credit card bill arrives or when we don't have such a good time at the party after all. But fashion magazines and the media encourage us to keep playing the game and many of us get hooked on it. One of our clients aptly referred to herself as a "fashion slave."

Of course, competition isn't always negative. There are many positive forms of competition, including competing with yourself. Getting through a challenging situation without compulsively eating or restricting yourself from food is one way to lovingly compete with yourself. Sports, hobbies, school work, etc., can all be positively or negatively competitive, depending on your motives. Ask yourself whether the activity is enjoyable and invigorating, or surrounded by fear and self-criticism.

Andrea's story about her relationship with exercise is an example of how she changed a negatively competitive experience into a positive one.

As a bona fide victim of the fitness industry, I spent countless years either forcing myself to exercise or beating myself up and bingeing when I didn't. I would go to the spa where I had a set routine based on the trend of the day. I would do the entire routine whether I wanted to or not. While exercising, I spent the majority of my time comparing myself to the other women, always feeling inadequate. I did love the feeling of a good workout, but I was so competitive and self-loathing that it ruined the positive feelings. When I got sick or injured, I became terrified. When I travelled, I would go to ridiculous lengths to be sure that I got my routine in. Again, if I didn't, I grew terrified. Such terror almost always led me to undereating or overeating.

One day, well into my recovery, I was on the treadmill and I looked around at others and asked myself, "What if my goal here was to be healthy rather than to lose weight?" I suddenly had the realization that exercise didn't have to be all about weight loss and drudgery and competing with people I knew nothing about. Exercise could be about health! What a novel idea! It felt like I had been in a prison and now a few of the bars were bent open.

This turning point led to many changes in the way I dealt with exercise. I became able to take a week off if I was sick or injured (without panicking, bingeing or dieting). I became able to loosen up on my set routine and listen more to my body's energy level. I began to look at the ways in which my body really wanted to move. And I finally began to let my body rest.

Today, my body's movement comes from my heart rather than my head. Last week I took a ballet class for the first time in 25 years (since the teacher told me I looked "chubby" in my tu-tu). Recently I found myself in the mood to run. In the mood? Who said that? Some days I want to hike briskly in the forest, other days I want to walk slowly and fully take in the scenery. Some days I arrive at the gym with the intention to work out, only to realize that I am tired. No longer fearing I will never exercise again, I promptly U-turn back home to spend the time curled up with a novel.

My relationship with exercise used to be uncomfortably competitive and fear-based. Today it is fun, balanced, self-loving, and joyful.

Fat Chat, unhealthy comparisons, excessive exercise, and fashion slavery all contain the belief that if we look better than other people, we will feel better about ourselves. But that's not true! People who seem "better" than us on the outside are not necessarily happier on the inside. Even "attractive" people have emotional pain. Andrea's story exemplifies this:

One of the lowest points in my life was when I was bingeing and vomiting several times a day. I was on my way to a support group meeting when I stopped at a gas station after a binge to vomit in the dirty public toilet bowl. I was especially humiliated because the food landed in the bowl so forcefully, toilet water and vomit splashed onto my face and hair.

In desperation, I proceeded to the support group. After I parked and got out of my car a woman from the group approached me and said, "I want to tell you how beautiful you are. I'm very jealous of you. You always seem so confident and together." I was stunned. "I have puke in my hair. I just binged and purged. How can you compare yourself to me?" I replied.

Now, many years later, after much healing and becoming a therapist, I see all kinds of women needlessly hating themselves and comparing themselves to others. Because I've been there, I know that the person they envy may be in just as much pain as they are.

So how do we change this tendency to compete, which destroys both our self-esteem and our relationships with other people? An alternative to competition is camaraderie. Letting go of competition and developing camaraderie means dropping out of the solo (me vs. them) "race" and joining a "team." There are many ways to join, and they all involve accepting ourselves and others as they are.

We can stop viewing ourselves and each other as the sum total of our external features and focus on getting to know who people are on the inside. We can stop participating in Fat Chat. The next time your friend says, "I'm so fat," you could say to her, "I'm learning that when I criticize my body I distract myself from deeper feelings. Do you want to talk about anything else that's going on for you?" And the next time you hear yourself starting to engage in Fat Chat, you can stop and ask yourself, "What am I actually feeling and needing right now? What would I be thinking about if I wasn't thinking about my body?"

We can join together and remind each other that the images of the models to whom we compare ourselves are often electronically altered — a computer may have erased or replaced parts of her body. We can acknowledge the life-threatening nutritional habits of supermodels and actresses. We can take into account that the same woman we are comparing ourselves to may feel lonely or unloved.

In the same way that talking to yourself in a negative manner never brings positive results, comparing yourself negatively to other people never brings positive results. Not only do these comparisons harm you, they also harm your relationships with others. While you're busy hating yourself and seeing others as better off, you are unavailable and distracted. You are probably also unable to acknowledge others' struggles, or to celebrate with them their joys and successes.

To counteract critical self-talk, we recommend that you to strive to achieve a balanced view of yourself, one wherein you accept your limitations (without shame), and honor your strengths (without putting others down).

To counteract unhealthy comparisons, we recommend *Well-Wishing*. Well-Wishing is thinking positively of other people, wishing for them the very best. While this can be challenging, it brings remarkable results — even if the person has no idea you're doing it!

Shelly, one of our clients, was having a conflict with a friend. After a few weeks of trying unsuccessfully to work it out, they gave up and stopped speaking to each other. Shelly felt much resentment and anger, and began to think negatively of her friend. Shelly admitted wishing bad things would happen, that her friend would regain the weight she'd lost, that everything wouldn't be so perfect in her friend's seemingly "perfect life." We introduced the concept of Well-Wishing to Shelly and she hated it! She realized, however, that resentment and anger were eating away at her, and that she was beginning to turn to food as a result. Shelly decided to try this new technique.

Each morning when Shelly woke up she wished that her friend would have a good day, be healthy, feel good, and have all the things Shelly wanted for herself. At first, she didn't believe any of this, didn't really want these things for her friend, but she kept wishing her well anyway. On the fifth day, Shelly ran into her friend in the supermarket. She strongly considered making a fast U-turn and going down a different aisle, but she didn't. Her friend greeted her with open arms. She was loving and apologetic and said she had been thinking about Shelly the past few days. Shelly and her friend made amends to each other right there. Shelly was amazed that after all her anger, she was able to be receptive to her friend's apology, and was even able to apologize herself. She was then aware that, in spite of her misgivings, her Well-Wishing had had a positive effect on her, reducing the time she spent fanning the flames of her anger. She realized, too, that in the past, she would have eaten and gained weight over the feud. Then she would have felt so poorly about herself, she would have definitely made that U-turn in the aisle and missed out on this healing experience.

Well-Wishing can be used with anyone, including strangers. When you notice yourself judging people by their looks, you can stop and wish them well. When you hear yourself gossiping about someone, you can wish them well instead. When you find yourself feeling jealous of someone, you can choose to wish that person well. Every time you do this, you are changing destructive thoughts into positive ones. When your thoughts are positive and noncompetitive, you will find yourself calmer and more content. And, of course, this will have a positive effect on your food choices, not to mention your overall health and well-being.

Hopefully, you have learned by now that the competitive mind-set can be a problem that stems from, and contributes to, low self-esteem, and leads to self-destructive eating. Another way to put an end to unhealthy competition is to become a better friend to yourself. This means honoring and taking care of yourself when you are thirsty, hungry or tired. This means dressing yourself comfortably and buying clothes that fit — no matter what size you are. It also means exercising (if you choose to) as a way to feel healthier and more energetic, not as a form of purging and punishment. Finally, it means honoring and taking care of your emotions.

Each of these actions requires you to listen to yourself. Remember the "part of you that knows?" (If not, see page 116.) This part knows when you need to exercise and when you need to rest, when you are uncomfortable, thirsty, needy, or content. It is your job to learn to listen to this part of yourself and take loving actions on your behalf. No one else can do this for you.

If we are to support each other, rather than compete, we can remind one another to consider our needs, to "check-in" with ourselves, to do what "the part of us that knows" is telling us we need to do. This may mean encouraging a friend who is exhausted to break her date with you (even though you really wanted to see her) so she can stay home and rest. Or it may mean encouraging her to come out with you anyway, because you know her desire to stay home is really about isolation, not self-care. Being a good friend means looking out for your friends' best interests while taking care of yourself. It means being honest, loving and respectful toward yourself and toward your friends.

To help us on our Journey toward self-acceptance and camaraderie, we need to develop a supportive circle of friends. Finding supportive friends of the same gender is especially important. Men need the companionship of men, just as women need the friendship of women. Each gender shares a unique perspective and communication style.

In recovery, our friendships with women are no longer focused on diets and exercise, what we eat, and what we look like. We now have deeply intimate relationships with our women friends, and we have men in our lives who know and love who we are, not just what we look like. Our friends know both our strengths and our weaknesses, and they support us in our self-care, as well as in our ongoing growth process.

The competitive drive to be as thin as, or as attractive as, other people only drives us apart from one another, separating us from friendship and love that might be available. When we accept ourselves as we are, and acknowledge others as they are, when we reach out to each other as friends rather than competitors, our Journey becomes easier and more relaxed. If you decide to drop out of the competitive "race," you'll find you have the opportunity to slow down and actually enjoy life.

Journey One

*Date:*_____

1. How much time would you guess you spend each week engaging in Fat Chat?

_____

2. How many times a day would you guess you make unhealthy comparisons between yourself and other people?

_____

3. How often do you engage in self-deprivation? Include depriving yourself of food, sleep, and any other form of self-care.

_____

4.   a. Make a list of people with whom you feel competitive or jealous, and write about why you feel this way with each of them:

_____
_____
_____
_____
_____

b. Write a kind wish for each of the people you just listed. If you can't think of a kind wish, wish for them something you wish for yourself, like peace of mind.

_____
_____
_____
_____
_____

c. What did it feel like to give kind wishes to these people?

_____

_____

_____

_____

_____

_____

5. Record below an accomplishment you recently shared with a friend, and the reaction you received. What was it like to share your accomplishment? If you haven't shared one recently, write about why you haven't; then write down the name of one person with whom you would be willing to share an accomplishment.

_____

_____

_____

_____

_____

6. Ask a friend what she feels good about in her life. Record below what she said, and the feelings in you that arose.

_____

_____

_____

_____

_____

7. Write about the amount of competition vs. the amount of supportive camaraderie you are currently experiencing in your life.

_____

_____

_____

_____

This sign designates what we will call a Spontaneous Road Trip. A Spontaneous Road Trip is akin to deciding to go off the beaten path and explore unknown territory. When you arrive at this sign in your workbook, we encourage you to do whatever you want on this page. You can use it to express anything going on for you at this time. You can draw, write spontaneously about your thoughts and feelings, make a collage, write a poem, insert a photograph of yourself... anything that will help you explore and record this current part of your Journey. (Remember there is no right or wrong way to do this!)

🌿 *Journey Two*

*Date:*_____

1. How much time would you guess you spend each week engaging in Fat Chat?

_____

2. How many times a day would you guess you make unhealthy comparisons between yourself and other women?

_____

3. How often do you engage in self-deprivation? Include depriving yourself of food, sleep, and any other form of self-care.

_____

4. Look back at your responses to the above three questions in Journey One. What do you notice?

_____
_____
_____
_____
_____
_____

5. How would you describe your relationship to exercise?

_____
_____
_____
_____
_____
_____

6.   a. List some qualities about yourself that you appreciate:

_____

_____

_____

_____

_____

_____

_____

_____

b. How does it feel to make such a list?

_____

_____

_____

_____

_____

_____

_____

_____

_____

_____

_____

❧ *Journey Three*

*Date:*_____

1. How much time would you guess you spend each week engaging in Fat Chat?

_____

2. How many times a day would you guess you make unhealthy comparisons between yourself and other women?

_____

3. How often do you engage in self-deprivation?

_____

4. Look back at your responses to the above three questions in Journeys One and Two. What do you notice?

_____

_____

_____

_____

_____

_____

_____

_____

_____

_____

_____

_____

_____

5. What is your relationship to exercise at this point in your Journey?

_____

_____

_____

_____

_____

6. How do you feel about the way you dress? Do you dress for comfort? Do you buy clothes that fit you? Do you hold onto clothes that no longer fit? Why or why not?

_____

_____

_____

_____

_____

_____

7. a. Write about the amount of competition vs. the amount of supportive camaraderie you are currently experiencing in your life.

_____

_____

_____

_____

_____

_____

b. Look back at this question in Journey One. What do you notice?

_____

_____

_____

_____

_____

_____

❧ *Journey Four*

*Date:*_____

1. With whom are you currently competitive?

_____

_____

_____

_____

_____

2. How are you affected by your competition with others?

_____

_____

_____

_____

_____

_____

3. What do you think would happen if you gave up competing with others and compared yourself only to yourself and how far you have come?

_____

_____

_____

_____

_____

_____

_____

_____

4. Pick someone from Question #1 above and write a well-wishing paragraph to them.

Dear_____, I wish for you . . .

_____

_____

_____

_____

_____

5. What feelings come up when you are well-wishing this person?

_____

_____

_____

_____

_____

6. Name some people with whom you feel a sense of camaraderie.

_____

_____

_____

_____

7. What feelings are you aware of as you look at the above list of people?

_____

_____

_____

_____

8. What are some of the things you now do in place of internal and external Fat Chat?

_____

_____

_____

_____

_____

Chapter 13

Holding On vs. Letting Go

People with food, weight and body image issues tend to hold on to things they would be better off letting go of, and to let go of things they would be better off holding on to. There is an appropriate time for holding on and an appropriate time for letting go. Usually, when we hold on inappropriately, or try to control, we do so out of fear. And no wonder. Letting go can feel terrifying. Rather than feeling the fear and frustration of being unable to control life events and other people, many of us distract ourselves by trying to control our eating and our weight. We take an intangible terror and make it into a tangible mission. The only trouble is that this doesn't work. If it did, none of us would be contending with ongoing body issues.

In order to surrender our control, we have to realize that control is really an illusion. There are more instances than most of us would like to admit over which we simply do not have control. Once we understand this, we often find that it's actually a relief to let go of control. Just realizing that we have the option of letting go can help us, in some cases, to feel less anxious. And, not only that — letting go often brings better results! If obsessing, or trying to control things, worked, or even helped, you would probably be thin, happy, and free by now.

We have worked with many clients who have struggled for years with an issue in their lives, trying every possible means of changing the situation or person. Finally, when they gave up trying to control it, and simply let go, the situation changed. This is because our desire to change someone or something creates tension and causes resistance. When people relax, they create room for change. We love this motto: "When nothing works, try doing nothing!"

Learning to trust the flow of life takes practice. Letting go doesn't mean being apathetic or neglectful. It means turning to your heart (the "part of you that knows"), and others (your support system), for guidance. The "part of you that knows" helps you act when needed, and hold back when inaction would be better. In day-to-day dealings it's okay to suggest to others ways to do something, but after the suggestion, it's up to them to do it or not. And it is up to you to let go (or not)! You can voice your opinions or feelings and you can do whatever you need to do to take care of yourself, but you can't control what other people actually do.

Ever notice that when you try to change someone, the person won't budge? Even if changing would obviously be in that person's best interests? Ever notice what happens when you let go? Often that's when the person begins to make changes, and, if not, at least you no longer waste your energy on an impossible task!

When it comes to romantic relationships, especially new ones, we often don't have the patience to let things unfold over time. Waiting, and not knowing the outcome, is too uncomfortable. From this place of fear and discomfort we try to manipulate and control what the relationship will be. We may insist on defining the relationship, or on having a commitment before the time is right. This often backfires and ends up sabotaging the relationship, rather than helping it. Relationships cannot be controlled.

Being in a relationship can be like traveling in a foreign country. If you do too much planning, you'll miss out on pleasant surprises and adventures. When you travel you may not know where you'll be stopping at the end of the day, but by staying open and present along the way, you are likely to see great scenery, meet interesting people, and enjoy the trip. In your relationships, if you try to control the outcome, you miss out on what is actually happening. And though you may feel safer when you attempt to control your relationships, you will most likely push people away and/or create conflicts. Letting relationships grow and unfold over time is hard, but it leaves room for spontaneity, true intimacy, and deep love.

Letting go of food and weight control can also lead you on some positive adventures. Most of us try to control our weight because we are terrified about what would happen if we didn't. We fail to see that it is our methods of control that are damaging, and that they aren't helping us to achieve what we really want — happiness and peace of mind. And when our methods of control don't work, we tend to blame ourselves or others, rather than our methods.

Because we have had problems controlling our eating, many of us see ourselves as weak-willed or lazy. Ironically, most of us tend to be very strong-willed. When our efforts to control don't work, we try to pull the reins even tighter. We hang in there far longer than is appropriate. We don't know when to let go. As a result, we sabotage the very things we want the most.

Andrea's experience of gradually learning to let go was key to her recovery:

> *Anything I write about letting go of my desire to lose weight seems like an understatement, given that I spent the majority of my life struggling to shrink my body. Without a doubt, losing weight was the most consistent goal I'd always had. Even after starting my recovery and learning about my emotions, my quest to lose weight, although it subsided, remained constant.*
>
> *I slowly lost weight over my first nine years in recovery (and incredibly, did not gain it back), but I still overate at times and struggled with my body size. I remember the day I decided to let go of the struggle. I was standing in front of a full-length mirror. I realized I had weighed the same amount, give or take five to ten pounds, for several years. Although I occasionally ate more than I needed, I was no longer bingeing, sneak-eating, or purging. Finally, I said to myself: "Can't this be good enough? Can't it be enough that I'm not bingeing every day?"*

I began to think that if weighing somewhat more than my "ideal" weight was the price I had to pay for eating freely and feeling sane around food, then it was a worthy price. I was not going to spend the second half of my life, as I had the first, battling with my body. Somehow — and I could not have arrived at this turning point a second before I did — I let go!

Then, without controlling it, or even being aware for the most part, I began to lose more weight. At times I found myself choosing not to eat simply because I wasn't hungry. The ability to do this came from the permission I had given myself to eat what and when I wanted, and from letting go of my anxiety around weight control.

Since it no longer mattered if I lost weight, I was free from the all-consuming anxiety about what I ate. I was finally faced with whether or not my body wanted food. There was no longer anything to rebel from, be "bad" about, or sabotage. People began noticing that I was losing weight, which was true, but the bigger truth was I had let go of losing weight.

Letting go is an elusive concept. However, there are some symbolic ways you can help yourself to do it. One way is to visualize what you want to let go of. This could be a person, a food, a situation, or even an unrealistic fantasy. Following is a Letting-Go Visualization. You may want to read it several times through to get the idea before trying it. You could also record it on a cassette tape, then do the exercise while listening to the tape. (Although this exercise doesn't make letting go happen in reality, it can give you much needed practice in feeling what it would be like to actually let go.)

Begin this letting-go process by closing your eyes and relaxing your body. (pause here) Take several deep breaths, in and out, focusing on breathing and relaxing. (long pause) Let your breathing return to normal. (pause here) Use your imagination now to picture a person or a situation that you are wanting to let go of. Picture the person or situation floating away like a leaf on a stream or drifting up into the sky inside a balloon. Use whatever image feels right for you. Stay with the scene until the person or situation is gone, allowing yourself to be aware of, and feel, all your responses as you watch the scene drift away.

One of our clients, Rebecca, uses visualization when she feels particularly stressed. She sits in a comfortable chair, closes her eyes and imagines that each stressful situation is inside a balloon. She pictures these balloons in different sizes, depending on how distressing each issue is. For example, she sees her financial worries as a very large balloon, and her deadline at work as a medium-sized one. After she sees a bouquet of balloons that includes every stressful issue, she imagines letting go of the bunch. In her mind's eye, she watches as the balloons drift into the sky, and get smaller and smaller until she can't see them. She says she feels lighter and relieved afterward. Though this exercise does not solve Rebecca's problems, she is grateful to have a tool that helps her have moments of letting go.

Another letting go activity involves making yourself a special can (also known as a Can-Let-Go-Can!) in which you deposit pieces of paper listing who and what you want to let go of. You can collage a coffee can or plastic canister using pictures or images that remind you of trusting and letting go. Every time you put a note in your Can-Let-Go-Can, you symbolize your intention to let go. Another client, Annette, uses her Can-Let-Go-Can every evening when she comes home from work. She writes down all the things that are bothering her, particularly situations she cannot control, folds up the paper and puts it in her can. As she does this, she says to herself, "I can let go," takes a deep breath, relaxes and lets go. Periodically, when Annette's can is filled, she takes out all the pieces of paper, puts them in her woodstove and burns them. Sometimes she reads them first, amazed that most of the situations have been resolved.

The art of letting go does not apply to everything. Knowing what to hold onto is also a crucial life skill. It's important to hold close to you things like praise, good memories, helpful friends and personal accomplishments. Too often, because we don't feel worthy, we discount, minimize, forget, and let go of these positive things. Letting go of the positive, and hanging on to the negative, keeps us forever dissatisfied and hungry. It is essential that we learn to acknowledge and hold on to what is good in our lives.

One example of positive holding on comes from a friend of ours who had cancer. Before going in for surgery, she held a gathering of her special women friends. She asked each woman to bring a small object that represented a strength they had used during a difficult time. Each person was invited to tell the story of their struggle and their strength. Then the women put all of their objects into a beautiful velvet pouch for their friend to bring with her to surgery. This ritual was her way of holding onto the strength and support of her friends while she went through a very challenging and frightening experience.

When we hold onto the positives, we increase our self-esteem and self-respect, and we reduce anxiety. We are better equipped to make decisions. With greater self-esteem and self-respect, it becomes easier to let go of things that contribute to feeling bad about ourselves, such as criticisms and judgments from other people. By holding onto, or valuing, our feelings and our truths, we become better able to work through difficult feelings, and eventually move on.

When we give up fighting and controlling, we often discover sadness or frustration that certain things are not going to go our way. These feelings are important to feel. We are better able to let go of these emotions when we have fully acknowledged and expressed them. Once that is done, letting go and moving on usually comes naturally.

Many people think that letting go is synonymous with giving up or losing. In our experience, it's more like going with the current, rather than fighting against it. You still get to swim, only it's a lot easier, and certainly more pleasant.

Surrendering does not necessarily mean sitting back and doing nothing. It means waiting until "the part of you that knows" is clear. Waiting can be difficult because sometimes it means being in transition and feeling confused or unresolved. We typically start obsessing on our weight when we are in these states. By letting go of the need for immediate resolution, and tuning into our hearts, our next steps will eventually become clear. This enables you to avoid acting impulsively out of fear and weakness. Instead, you act calmly from wisdom and strength, letting go of what doesn't work and holding on to what does.

❧ *Journey One*

*Date:*_____

1. As a physical example of holding on, try holding your breath for 10 seconds, then letting it go. What are you aware of when you hold your breath? What are you aware of when you let it go?

_____

_____

_____

_____

_____

2. Who in the past have you tried to control, and what happened?

_____

_____

_____

_____

_____

3. Who are you currently trying to control, and what is happening as a result?

_____

_____

_____

_____

_____

4. Who or what do you need to let go of? Why?

_____

_____

_____

_____

5. Complete the following sentences:

    a. I'm afraid if I let go of trying to control _____ then . . .

    b. I'm afraid if I don't let go of trying to control _____ then . . .

6. What are some good things in your life that you have not been acknowledging?

_____

_____

_____

_____

_____

_____

_____

7. How do you feel as you think about positive things in your life?

_____

_____

_____

_____

_____

_____

_____

_____

_____

_____

_____

❧ *Journey Two*

*Date:*_____

1. Complete the following letter:
   Dear Food and Weight Obsession:
   In order to let you go I need to . . .

   _____

   _____

   _____

   _____

   _____

   _____

2.   a. Describe what you are scared about, and detail how you try to control those situations.

   _____

   _____

   _____

   _____

   _____

   b. What works and what doesn't work about your current approaches?

   _____

   _____

   _____

3. Remember a time in the past when you let go and the situation improved. What happened?

   _____

   _____

   _____

   _____

   _____

4. Pick one thing you are willing to let go of, if only a little bit. Write it down. Name one small step you can take in letting it go.

_____

_____

_____

_____

_____

5. What comfort or truths do you need to hold onto, or remember, right now?

For example, "I need to hold onto the knowledge that many people love me," or "I need to remember the positive feedback my employer gave me today."

_____

_____

_____

_____

_____

_____

6. What are some good things in your life that you have not been acknowledging?

_____

_____

_____

_____

_____

_____

7. How do you feel as you think about positive things in your life?

_____

_____

_____

_____

_____

❧ *Journey Three*

*Date:*_____

1. Look back at Journey One, Question #4. Were you able to let go of that person or situation? If so, what happened? If not, what happened?

_____
_____
_____
_____
_____
_____
_____

2. Look back at Journey Two, Question #4. Did you take that step? If so, what happened? If not, what happened?

_____
_____
_____
_____
_____
_____
_____

3. What or who are you trying to control right now? How effective are you?

_____
_____
_____
_____
_____

4. What would you be willing to let go of? How could you do that?

_____

_____

_____

_____

_____

_____

_____

_____

_____

5. What are some positive things in your life you can acknowledge?

_____

_____

_____

_____

_____

_____

_____

_____

_____

6. Look back at Journeys One and Two, Questions #6 and #7. What do you notice about your ability to acknowledge yourself then, verses your ability to do so now?

_____

_____

_____

_____

_____

_____

❧ *Journey Four*

*Date:*_____

1. List all the things you would like to let go of.

_____

_____

_____

_____

_____

_____

_____

_____

2. Write below some of the evidence you have that you cannot control the things you listed above.

_____

_____

_____

_____

_____

_____

_____

_____

3. Now think of three tangible ways you can assist yourself in letting go.

_____

_____

_____

_____

_____

_____

4. What are some things you need to hold onto?

_____

_____

_____

_____

_____

_____

5. Draw a picture of yourself illustrating what you would look like if you let go of all you wish to be rid of, while holding onto all you need.

6. Make as long a list as you possibly can of your skills, gifts, and accomplishments. (If you have trouble making a list, write anything you can think of and add to the list later as you remember more.)

_____

_____

_____

_____

_____

_____

This sign designates what we will call a Spontaneous Road Trip. A Spontaneous Road Trip is akin to deciding to go off the beaten path and explore unknown territory. When you arrive at this sign in your workbook, we encourage you to do whatever you want on this page. You can use it to express anything going on for you at this time. You can draw, write spontaneously about your thoughts and feelings, make a collage, write a poem, insert a photograph of yourself... anything that will help you explore and record this current part of your Journey. (Remember there is no right or wrong way to do this!)

Chapter 14

Human Doing vs. Human Being

Maintaining an active, diverse lifestyle is healthy. But too much activity can keep us from living a balanced life or distract us from issues that need our attention. Just as food can divert us from our feelings, so too can "busyness." Sometimes we avoid our feelings by alternating between out-of-control eating and out-of-control doing. Many people don't know how to slow down and rest, aside from tranquilizing themselves with food. Often people escape troubling emotions by frenetically engaging in one activity after another. We usually don't do this consciously, but our cultural work ethic encourages such a pattern, which can then become a way of life.

The same low self-esteem that contributes to food, weight and body image issues can also motivate a hectic lifestyle. Many people feel they can't justify resting or simply being; they feel compelled toward constant doing. It is simply untrue that busyness justifies one's existence! Just by virtue of being alive, you have a right to be here. You have a right to enjoy life and to use at least some of your time to nurture yourself. You have a right, and a need, to relax. You have a right to do nothing sometimes.

Here is Andrea's story about becoming comfortable with herself whether she was busy or not.

> After many years of working at a counseling agency and slowly trying to build my psychotherapy practice on the side, I finally decided to take the plunge into a full-time private practice. At first there were days when I had few or no clients. This meant that I had a lot of unstructured time. On these days, I felt horrible about myself. I believed I should be doing something at all times, that I should be busy, accomplishing things. I also felt panicked about being able to support myself. I would check my phone messages constantly. On particularly slow days, when Michael would come home from work and ask me what I had done that day, I would either snap at him,

invent some important errands to try to justify my existence, or burst into tears and tell him I felt worthless and hadn't gotten out of my robe all day.

As I continued to use my support system to express and come to terms with my feeling of worthlessness, I saw that I did not have to constantly be doing or accomplishing in order to be okay. I was loved and worthy of love no matter how I filled my day.

Over time, my schedule has become much more balanced. During my free time I have learned to let myself do what I feel like doing. I no longer make up excuses, tell myself I'm worthless, or panic about money. Today, doing absolutely nothing is just as valuable to me as a full day of work.

It is challenging for people with food, weight, and body image issues to slow down and live in the present. Often, the present is not where we want to be because there are things about it that we don't like, and feelings that we don't want to feel. Worrying about the future (which is one way to not be present) seems safer. We tend to think that if we worry about the future, we will be able to improve it. However, even though some of us make a full-time job out of it, worrying is a useless act. Most of what we worry about never happens! Worrying is an endless task because there are an infinite combination of concerns over which one can obsess. Worrying about what will happen in the future does not help us cope with what is happening today, and it makes today miserable. Instead of worrying, we can learn to problem-solve, seek out help, vent our fears, and let the future naturally unfold. When we learn to let go of our worrying, we give ourselves the opportunity to deal with how things are, rather than how we think they should be.

The present moment is filled with many challenges, such as: how to feel good about ourselves right now, how to discover what we need right now (e.g. nurturing, companionship, rest) and finding ways to get our needs met. Developing and working toward future goals is important, but it is the present that matters most in terms of how we actually experience our lives. Do we have clarity right now, or lack of clarity? Do we have emotional intimacy in our lives today, or lack of emotional intimacy? Do we feel connected to ourselves and others, or disconnected? These are questions that, if attended to now, will positively impact our future.

Slowing down and spending time being present does not mean that we will do nothing, although at times it might. It means we take the time for our motivation to come from the "part of us that knows," rather than from our fears and our "shoulds." When we tune in to "the part of us that knows" we find out exactly what is best for us to do at any given moment. Sometimes we need to get things done, and sometimes we need to relax and slow down. We are most healthy, clear, and alert when these are balanced. It is helpful to regularly ask yourself, "What do I need to do to take care of myself right now?"

Doing, in itself, is not a bad thing. It is only when we go overboard and do too much, or do things in a compulsive manner, that doing becomes self-destructive. In fact, there are many things you can do that can aide you in connecting with yourself and learning to be. Here is a list of things that we have done that have helped us to connect with ourselves, and also with the "part of us that knows."

Meditation
Prayer
Visualization
Affirmations (positive statements about yourself)
Mantras (repeating a loving word or phrase)
Deep breathing
Reading inspirational books
Listening to music
Writing

One client of ours, named Mindy, realized that much of her overeating was about past sadness and anger, and anxiety about her future. She realized she was rarely in the present. While running errands, she felt frantic and out-of-control, as if she was being "chased." She knows now that she can stop when her day feels frenetic and ask herself, "What am I afraid of right now?" She says it's usually something about her past or future, and once she gives herself time to identify what it is and get the appropriate support, she can resume her chores without feeling frantic, or turning to food.

Early on in this process, it may be difficult for you to slow down and be still. That's okay. Five seconds is better than none! You can slowly build from there as your tolerance for experiencing your emotions increases. What often makes it hard to slow down is that we fear the feelings and judgments that may arise when we do so. For this reason, it may be helpful to do some writing as part of your effort to relax. Writing itself may not be relaxing, but it is a good way to begin the slowing down process and discharge the feelings that arise when you attempt to relax.

As challenging as it may seem, it can be a liberating experience to allow yourself an unplanned day (or an hour, or even 15 minutes!) to slow down and do as you please. Letting up on the schedules that run your life might mean that you won't get everything done, but at least you'll enjoy what you do. Even after a nonstop busy day, have you ever noticed how there is always more to do? Another errand is always waiting to distract us from ourselves. Take laundry, for example. While you are getting your laundry done, the clothes you are wearing are getting dirty! There is always more to do. It's up to you to create break time.

In many cases we create our own anxiety through excessive list-making and over-commitment. These habits keep us in a perpetual state of anxiety, guilt, and worry. Many of us have an unconscious belief that if we get all our errands, chores, and lists completed, we'll finally feel okay. But getting everything done will not fix you! Besides, we rarely get everything done anyway. Though a checked-off errand list may give you some feeling of accomplishment, it won't heal a self-esteem problem.

If, however, you need to make a list, and you're the kind of person who thinks you have to get it all done today, what about changing your list of "things to do today," to a list of "things to do this week" (or this month)? If you're the kind of person who never finds time for yourself no matter what, try developing a "What I'd Really Like to Do" list. Then, actually create time for these enjoyable endeavors. Many of our clients are incredibly giving people — to everyone but themselves. What would it take for you to put yourself on the list of important people in your life?

We encourage you to talk back to that critical voice in your head that constantly pushes you. Tell it you deserve to take a rest. We know there are many necessities in life that must be done, but at some point everybody deserves to rest! Stopping for a few seconds, even if it's just to notice your busyness and the fear that underlies it, is an important first step. Other short stops include taking a long deep breath, pausing to look out the window for a minute, or closing your eyes and picturing your favorite peaceful place. Learning to take longer breaks is also an essential skill on your Journey. Such breaks might include: lying on the couch (without food), walking in the sunshine, listening to a relaxation tape, taking a bath or a hot tub.

Life is not an emergency! Although your life may be full of necessary responsibilities, there is still time for finding a few moments to simply be. Even one minute of stopping goes a long way.

Journey One

Date:_____

1. Close your eyes and sit quietly for 30 seconds. Notice what comes up. Are the thoughts and feelings from your past, present, or future?

_____

_____

_____

_____

_____

2. Looking back on your day today, what motivated your activities? Were you motivated by fear? Were you motivated by "the part of you that knows?" How did you decide what to do today?

_____

_____

_____

_____

_____

3.   a. What are you worrying about?

_____

_____

_____

_____

    b. Which concerns in the above list are actually happening in the present?

_____

_____

_____

_____

4.   a. How much unstructured time did you have this past week?

_____

   b. How did you handle it?

_____

_____

_____

_____

   c. What would help you to handle it better?

_____

_____

_____

_____

   d. If you didn't have any unstructured time, what would help you create some?

_____

_____

_____

_____

_____

_____

5. What do you need to do to take care of yourself right now?

_____

_____

_____

_____

_____

_____

🌿 *Journey Two*

*Date:*_____

1. Make a list of the things that are worrying you. Beside each concern note whether the worry belongs in the past, present, or future.

_____

_____

_____

_____

_____

_____

_____

_____

2. What will happen if you don't get everything done that you think you should?

_____

_____

_____

_____

_____

_____

_____

3.   a. Practice being present for three minutes. Afterwards, write down everything you saw, heard, smelled, thought, and felt.

_____

_____

_____

_____

_____

b. What was it like to do that?

_____

_____

_____

4.   a. List some times when you found yourself compulsively busy this week.

_____

_____

_____

_____

b. What do you think triggered you to get into a compulsive mode? What do you think you might have felt if you had let yourself be still?

_____

_____

_____

_____

5.   a. List some times when you were busy this week, but did not feel compulsive.

_____

_____

_____

_____

b. How does compulsive busyness feel different from healthy busyness?

_____

_____

_____

_____

6. What do you need to do to take care of yourself right now?

_____

_____

_____

This sign designates what we call a Spontaneous Road Trip. A Spontaneous Road Trip is akin to deciding to go off the beaten path and explore unknown territory. When you arrive at this sign in your workbook, we encourage you to do whatever you want on this page. You can use it to express anything going on for you at this time. You can draw, write spontaneously about your thoughts and feelings, make a collage, write a poem, insert a photograph of yourself... anything that will help you explore and record this current part of your Journey. (Remember there is no right or wrong way to do this!)

❧ *Journey Three*

*Date:*_____

1. Make note of what motivated your different activities today. Were you being propelled by fear or peacefulness?

_____

_____

_____

_____

2.   a. How much unstructured time did you have this past week?

_____

   b. How did you handle it?

_____

_____

_____

   c. Look back on Journey One, Question #4. How does the way you handle unstructured time now compare to then?

_____

_____

_____

_____

3. What situations in your life, if attended to, would make it easier for you to slow down and be more comfortable with yourself?

_____

_____

_____

_____

_____

4. a. Practice being present for three minutes. Afterwards, write down everything you saw, heard, smelled, thought, and felt.

_____

_____

_____

_____

_____

b. What was it like to do that?

_____

_____

_____

_____

c. Look back at Journey Two, Question #3. What changes do you notice in your ability to be present?

_____

_____

_____

_____

_____

5. Who are the people that you put ahead of yourself? Is this appropriate? If yes, is there ever a time when it's not?

_____

_____

_____

_____

6. What do you need to do to take care of yourself right now?

_____

_____

_____

_____

🌺 *Journey Four*

Date:_____

1. Looking back on your day today, what motivated your activities? Were you motivated by fear? Were you motivated by the "part of you that knows?" How did you decide what to do today?

_____

_____

_____

_____

_____

_____

2. Look back at Journey One, Questions #2 though #4. What has changed in how you handle your days?

_____

_____

_____

_____

_____

3. Write about the feelings and thoughts that normally arise when you slow down or rest (without food).

_____

_____

_____

_____

4. Of what do you need to remind yourself in order for you to be able to slow down, rest, or take a break, without berating yourself?

_____

_____

_____

_____

5. Plan a time in the next week (or two) when you can give yourself unstructured time to use in whatever way seems appropriate. Write here the day and time, and also mark it on your calendar.

_____

6. Describe what the unstructured time was like, and what thoughts or feelings arose as you experienced it.

_____
_____
_____
_____
_____
_____

7. If you didn't arrange for some free time, write about what stopped you, and the feelings that you have about it.

_____
_____
_____
_____
_____
_____
_____

8. What do you need to do to take care of yourself right now?

_____
_____
_____
_____
_____
_____
_____

Chapter 15

Endings vs. Beginnings

How many times have you read a self-help book, joined a health spa, signed up for a diet, and vowed this was the beginning of a "new you?" Then, a few weeks later, you quit it all and were back to your "old self" and old habits. The Live-It approach can make finishing this book a very different experience for you. Changing how you relate to food, people, your emotions, and your body is an ongoing process with many ups and downs. A Live-It is not all-or-nothing and it does not end. If you hurt yourself with food yesterday, it does not mean you "blew it" and need to "start over" today. It means you had difficulty coping with something in your life yesterday and today you can seek help in finding a better way to cope.

Therefore, the end of this book, no matter where you are in your recovery process, is an opportunity for a new beginning. Rather than judging yourself, and deciding you haven't done it good enough, we encourage you to praise yourself for making it this far and to keep going. We have included four Journeys in this book, because we know it can take that many, or more, to absorb all this information and actually make changes.

You now have techniques to practice, like Rainbow Thinking, Loving Limits, and Loving Confrontation. If you have a conflict with a friend, it doesn't mean you have to end the relationship. Now you can get support in dealing with the conflict and find ways to develop deeper relationships. And if you are feeling badly about your body, we hope you now know that the solution is not in changing your body. It's in finding out what feelings led you to this distracting obsession, and learning to nourish your emotional self instead.

All endings and beginnings involve change. Coping with the emotions brought on by change takes both practice and patience. Even when the change is positive! Every change, even one for the better, involves loss, and most changes also involve some degree of fear. Feelings of fear and sadness must be experienced and addressed if we are to make healthy transitions. If we ignore, avoid or deny these emotions, we find ourselves overeating and/or obsessing about our bodies again. It's important to acknowledge when you are in the midst of a change, so that you can cope with the myriad of feelings that come along with it.

When we talk about change, we can talk about big changes such as death, divorce, birth, or a move. We can also talk about the smaller daily changes, like transitioning from work to home, from being in a group to being alone, from napping to waking up. Even small changes such as these can evoke feelings from which we can easily turn away. Rather than recognize the transition and the difficult feelings, many of us immediately turn to food, not even knowing why. Somehow it seems easier to divert our focus to a particular food, a bowl, a bag, the freezer, or the stove. Often just naming and sitting with the feelings for a few minutes is enough for them to pass. But we are people who have had little tolerance for our emotions and find it difficult to wait for even one minute.

Along your Journey of Recovery, as well as throughout your life, there will be many endings and beginnings. Not all of these will be external changes. Some will be internal, as you change how you think and how you attend to your feelings. All change brings feelings.

We used to think that once we lost weight, our problems would be over. Instead, we found that as we began to focus on, and feel our feelings, we actually felt worse at times! This is because, after years of stuffing our feelings, when we finally allow them to emerge, they feel uncomfortable and overwhelming. After all, if we were comfortable with our emotions, we wouldn't have stuffed them down in the first place! Overeating was a more familiar, and therefore, more tolerable pain, than the pain of grief and loss.

In the early stages of recovery, you do feel better. That is, you feel everything better! You feel emotions you never even knew you had. The power of feelings is what makes the Journey so challenging, and why many people end up overeating or dieting again. It is crucial to have support and reassurance from people who have been where you are, and who have learned to live with their feeling selves. Without safe people to help you through your transitions, food is likely to become your support. Appendix A offers a resource list for finding support on your Journey.

Good-byes are a difficult type of change, and many people handle them poorly. One typical way people avoid painful good-byes is to manufacture a fight or a disagreement. Under the guise of fighting, we avoid the real feelings of sadness. We substitute anger (and probably eating) instead.

Another way of denying a good-bye, or a change, is to purposely avoid people from whom we are separating. While this can seem to spare some pain, the pain is still there, and on top of that, the relationship is without resolution.

While some people end relationships too abruptly, others cling to someone or something that needs to end. They are unwilling to face the change and the feelings it will bring. Many of us stay in relationships far too long because we don't know how to deal with the pain of letting go and the grief that would follow, even if the change would be positive.

Life is constantly changing, full of beginnings and endings. But sometimes we instigate unnecessary changes due to fears of closeness or abandonment. Safe people and the "part of you that knows" can assist you in distinguishing between a natural change that is healthy, sane, necessary or unavoidable, and one that comes out of fear or a desire to avoid feelings. With some preparation, saying good-bye can be an intimate, creative and even positive experience. Next time you see a good-bye coming, try to acknowledge the feelings and share them with the person from whom you are parting, and with other supportive people, or both.

There are many feelings that may come up when someone is leaving. Sometimes people feel angry that they are losing a companion, sometimes people are scared because they don't know what the changes will bring. Often, a good-bye will trigger feelings left over from previous good-byes — especially if we stuffed, rather than felt, those feelings at the time.

One way to have a healthy good-bye is to create a ritual that will make a special memory of your farewell. Good-bye parties are one way to honor a final meeting. Writing a good-bye letter and reflecting on the past and future, as well as on the happy and sad feelings, can be an excellent vehicle for bringing things to a graceful closure.

Marsea's story about how she handled two relocations at different times in her life offers insight on good-byes:

> *Before recovery, when I was dieting and bingeing and not aware of my feelings, I had to make a move. I had been living for a few years with two housemates whom I really liked. I was scared of my feelings, and of theirs as well. So rather than inform them of the move and allow time for their reactions, I wound up creating conflict with them and leaving suddenly without any good-byes. I was completely unaware of doing this at the time, but looking back now, I see it was easier for me to leave hating them, than missing them. I don't remember what our big argument was about, but I do remember being out-of-control with my eating during this transition. Years later, when I understood my feelings and actions better, I tracked down those old housemates and apologized. By doing that, I created a new and better ending for all of us.*

> *More recently, I faced another move. This time I made a big deal about it. I gave all my friends plenty of notice that I'd be going and tried to complete my involvements. I had several little going-away parties. I made time to hang out with people, to tell them what they meant to me, and to give them opportunities to express their feelings about my leaving. I'd listen even if they were upset or mad, which several people were. I allowed myself to recognize that these people really loved me and would miss my presence. I also took time to write about the various feelings I had. Although I was excited about the move, I didn't ignore the sadness I felt. And even though I knew the move was the right thing for me to do, I let myself feel the fear about leaving behind all that was familiar. To ease my transition, I made plans for Andrea to be with me my first weekend in the new city. She was my "safe person" who was there for me through all the different emotions I was going through. You can probably guess the ending of this story: I didn't overeat, and I didn't starve or deprive myself. In fact, food wasn't even an issue! Pretty amazing for someone who ate her way through every good-bye for the first 30 years of her life!*

Other lessons in how to say good-bye come from the support groups we lead. During the 16-week course of these groups, participants often become very close. Taking time to acknowledge the group's ending is very important. Encouraging the group members to express their feelings and their plans, and to review the value and the shortcomings of the group, are all part of a good-bye process. Having them take the time to clear up any concerns or questions they've had, or have been keeping from each other, also paves the way for clean, healthy good-byes. One group exercise is so obvious it could easily be overlooked. It is the actual act of saying "Good-bye." Just the word itself evokes strong feelings. People in the groups often try to avoid it by saying things like, "I'm sure we'll see each other again. We don't need to say good-bye." But the truth is that when a group ends, relationships change. So we encourage them to say "good-bye" and to allow themselves the feeling of sadness that "good-bye" evokes. Truly feeling the feelings about the ending is the first step toward a new beginning.

The good-bye that comes with a death is perhaps the most difficult of life's experiences. Such a major event often triggers abuse of food or other substances, weight obsession, or a plunge into depression. By paying attention to, and expressing all the feelings associated with, a death, severe depression and/or overeating can be avoided or lessened. Many of us censor our emotions, judging them as inappropriate, or too much for others to handle. This does not benefit us, it only interrupts our grieving and healing processes. If the people around us can't handle our grief, we need to find people who can. They are out there.

It is never too late to have a conscious closure with someone, even if they have been dead or gone for a long time. You can write a final good-bye letter, go to a special place where you can remember them, and say good-bye. Or you can create a special memorial for them in your house. The options are endless for consciously honoring your need to feel and express your grief and to say good-bye to someone who was important to you (even if they were important in a negative or painful way).

Few good-byes are as dramatic as death. But there are turning points sprinkled throughout our lives. Each involves a beginning and an ending: entering kindergarten, going to summer camp, graduating from high school and college, starting a new job, breaking up a relationship, moving to a new neighborhood or town, getting married, having children, having your children leave home, changing careers, or making changes in your life such as the ones represented by your work in this workbook. Every change brings a good-bye. Developing ways to experience and express all these good-byes will help you make healthy transitions from endings to new beginnings.

Throughout this workbook, we have presented you with many new concepts and tools with which to heal your food and weight problems. But it is not enough to just read about them. It is essential that you put them into practice. At the end of this chapter, you will find a checklist that will help you assess your progress after each Journey.

We know that each and every one of you has your own pace for healing. We also know that the people who actually practice the suggestions in this book — the people who courageously break their isolation and reach out to safe people, the people who take the risk to practice assertive communication, the people who push past their defenses and express the pain that is buried inside — experience more relief and freedom than those who just read this book and put it on the shelf. Your food and weight issues have been with you for a long time and they will not easily disappear. It will take effort and perseverance. Consider using even a quarter of the effort you have put into losing weight!

We understand that it may take a few times going through this book before you can put some of the concepts into practice. For this reason, we have provided you with four different Journeys to work on. So the ending of this workbook, right now, also signifies an opportunity for a new beginning. We hope you will reread each chapter, and then follow it with the next set of Journey questions. Many people find that when they read the chapters for a second, third, and even fourth time, they discover ideas that they hadn't noticed when they first read the book. As recovery progresses, they become less numb and find they are able to integrate more of what they are reading. They also find that the continuous reminders of what it takes to recover help them to finally act in ways that in the beginning seemed impossible to do.

A final note of hope from Marsea and Andrea:

We want you to know that it is possible to heal from the prison of food and weight pain. When we began our Journeys we had no idea that underneath the weight obsession and daily bingeing was a wellspring of painful emotions. And who knew that dealing with those emotions would lead us to our creativity, passions, and joy?

It is possible for you to recover from your food and weight pain, to find and heal what you have been eating over and running from. We welcome you to your next Journey, we applaud you for getting this far, and we cheer you on as you continue toward health and find what you've been hungry for all along.

This sign designates what we will call a Spontaneous Road Trip. A Spontaneous Road Trip is akin to deciding to go off the beaten path and explore unknown territory. When you arrive at this sign in your workbook, we encourage you to do whatever you want on this page. You can use it to express anything going on for you at this time. You can draw, write spontaneously about your thoughts and feelings, make a collage, write a poem, insert a photograph of yourself . . . anything that will help you explore and record this current part of your Journey. (Remember there is no right or wrong way to do this!)

Journey One Checkpoint

Check your progress for each of the following necessary components for recovery.

	no progress	some progress	significant progress	no longer an issue
Reaching out to safe people				
Identifying feelings				
Expressing feelings				
Assertive Communication				
Self-praise/compassion				
Rainbow Thinking				
Loving Limits				
Distinguishing between emotional and physical hunger				
Defining your Live-It				
Listening to your body				
Freedom from food and weight obsession				
Accepting your body				
Camaraderie				
Relaxing				
Connecting with "the part of you that knows"				
Letting go of control				

Goals for Journey Two:

1. _____
2. _____
3. _____

For example: 1. Become clearer about my Live-It
2. Learn how to meditate
3. Get help learning to be assertive with my mother

Journey One

*Date:*_____

1.   a. What endings does this time mark for you?

_____

_____

_____

_____

      b. What beginnings?

_____

_____

_____

_____

2. What feelings do you associate with the above endings and beginnings?

_____

_____

_____

_____

_____

_____

3. What are some of the things you learned about yourself during your Journey One experience through this book?

_____

_____

_____

_____

_____

_____

4. Which chapter have you incorporated the most into your life?

_____

5. Which chapter are you struggling with the most? Why?

_____

_____

_____

_____

_____

_____

_____

6. Use the space below to praise yourself for completing this Journey, even if you think you did it "imperfectly."

_____

_____

_____

_____

_____

_____

_____

_____

7. What are the next steps in your recovery process?

_____

_____

_____

_____

_____

_____

Journey Two Checkpoint

Check your progress for each of the following necessary components for recovery.

	no progress	some progress	significant progress	no longer an issue
Reaching out to safe people				
Identifying feelings				
Expressing feelings				
Assertive Communication				
Self-praise/compassion				
Rainbow Thinking				
Loving Limits				
Distinguishing between emotional and physical hunger				
Defining your Live-It				
Listening to your body				
Freedom from food and weight obsession				
Accepting your body				
Camaraderie				
Relaxing				
Connecting with "the part of you that knows"				
Letting go of control				

Goals for Journey Three:

1. _____
2. _____
3. _____

For example: 1. Become clearer about my Live-It

2. Learn how to meditate

3. Get help learning to be assertive with my mother

❧ *Journey Two*

*Date:*_____

1. Write down a history of good-byes you have made. Include farewells to friends, school, camp, homes, or anything that comes to mind. How did you handle those farewells? Do you notice any patterns?

_____

_____

_____

_____

_____

_____

_____

_____

_____

_____

2. Are there any good-byes that feel unfinished for you? Which ones?

_____

_____

_____

_____

_____

3. Write below, all the feelings associated with these unfinished good-byes.

_____

_____

_____

_____

_____

_____

4. Are there actions or rituals you could perform to bring these good-byes to closure, e.g.: write a good-bye letter, poem, or story? Other ideas are spending time with the person and talking about your unfinished feelings, sharing your feelings with a different (safe) person, playing a song that reminds you of the person, and allowing yourself to cry and really miss them, and then to say good-bye. Write something you are willing to do.

_____

_____

_____

_____

_____

5. What are some things you learned about yourself through your experience of Journey Two?

_____

_____

_____

_____

_____

6. Use the space below to praise yourself for completing this Journey, even if you think you did it "imperfectly."

_____

_____

_____

_____

_____

7. What might be your next steps on your Journey of Recovery?

_____

_____

_____

_____

_____

Journey Three Checkpoint

Check your progress for each of the following necessary components for recovery.

	no progress	some progress	significant progress	no longer an issue
Reaching out to safe people				
Identifying feelings				
Expressing feelings				
Assertive Communication				
Self-praise/compassion				
Rainbow Thinking				
Loving Limits				
Distinguishing between emotional and physical hunger				
Defining your Live-It				
Listening to your body				
Freedom from food and weight obsession				
Accepting your body				
Camaraderie				
Relaxing				
Connecting with "the part of you that knows"				
Letting go of control				

Goals for Journey Four:

1. _____
2. _____
3. _____

For example: 1. Become clearer about my Live-It
2. Learn how to meditate
3. Get help learning to be assertive with my mother

Journey Three

Date:____________________________

1. How did/do the people in your family handle good-byes, beginnings and transitions?

2. On a separate piece of paper, write a good-bye letter to a person, or several people in your past, to whom you didn't finish saying good-bye. Write here what it felt like to do that.

3. Select an aspect of food, your weight or your body image that you are willing to say good-bye to and, in whatever way feels right to you, use the space below to express your good-bye (i.e. letter, poem, drawing, collage, story). For example, you can say good-bye to your scale, to dieting, to overeating, to purging, to self-criticism or to any other self-destructive behavior.

4. What good-byes are you currently facing? What are your plans for honoring all the feelings that will accompany your upcoming good-byes?

_____

_____

_____

_____

_____

_____

5. What did you learn about yourself in Journey Three?

_____

_____

_____

_____

_____

_____

6. Use the space below to praise yourself for completing this Journey, even if you think you did it "imperfectly."

_____

_____

_____

_____

_____

_____

7. What are your plans for continuing your Journey of Recovery?

_____

_____

_____

_____

_____

_____

Journey Four Checkpoint

Check your progress for each of the following necessary components for recovery.

	no progress	some progress	significant progress	no longer an issue
Reaching out to safe people				
Identifying feelings				
Expressing feelings				
Assertive Communication				
Self-praise/compassion				
Rainbow Thinking				
Loving Limits				
Distinguishing between emotional and physical hunger				
Defining your Live-It				
Listening to your body				
Freedom from food and weight obsession				
Accepting your body				
Camaraderie				
Relaxing				
Connecting with "the part of you that knows"				
Letting go of control				

❧ *Journey Four*

Date:_____

1.   a. What endings does this time mark for you?

_____

_____

_____

_____

_____

b. What beginnings?

_____

_____

_____

_____

_____

2. What feelings do you associate with the above endings and beginnings?

_____

_____

_____

_____

_____

3. Describe a time when you avoided dealing with an ending. How did you avoid it? What happened as a result of your avoidance?

_____

_____

_____

_____

4. Describe a time when you obtained closure with something that ended. What provided the closure? What happened as a result of having closure?

_____

_____

_____

_____

_____

_____

_____

_____

5. To whom or what do you need to say good-bye to right now?

_____

_____

_____

_____

_____

_____

6. List some possible ways you can create closure.

_____

_____

_____

_____

_____

_____

_____

_____

7. What are some of the things you learned about yourself throughout your experience of Journey Four?

_____

_____

_____

_____

_____

_____

_____

_____

_____

_____

8. Use the space below to praise yourself for completing this workbook, even if you think you did it "imperfectly."

_____

_____

_____

_____

_____

_____

_____

9. What are some things you are going to do to continue your Journey of Recovery?

_____

_____

_____

_____

_____

_____

_____

_____

_____

_____

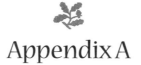

Appendix A

National Non-Profit Organizations

ACADEMY FOR EATING DISORDERS
6728 Old McLean Dr.
McLean, VA 22101
(703) 556-9222
www.acadeatdis.org
An association of multidisciplinary professionals; promotes effective treatment, develops prevention initiatives, advocates for the field, stimulates research, sponsors conferences.

AMERICAN ANOREXIA/BULIMIA ASSOCIATION
165 West 46th St. #1108
New York, NY 10036
(212) 575-6200
http://members.aol.com/AmanBu
A source of public information, support groups, referral speakers, educational programs, professional training, and a quarterly newsletter.

NATIONAL ASSOCIATION OF ANOREXIA NERVOSA AND ASSOCIATED DISORDERS
P.O. Box 7
Highland Park, IL 60035
(708) 831-3438
www.members.aol.com/anad20
Distributes listing of therapists, hospitals, and informative materials; sponsors support groups, conferences, advocacy campaigns, research and a crisis hot line.

EATING DISORDERS AWARENESS AND PREVENTION
603 Stewart St. # 803
Seattle, WA 98101
(206) 382-3587
www.members.aol.com/edapinc/home.html
Sponsors Eating Disorders Awareness Week in February with a network of state coordinators and educational programs.

INTERNATIONAL ASSOCIATION OF EATING DISORDER PROFESSIONALS
427 Whooping Loop #1819
Altamonte Springs, FL 32701
(800) 800-8126
www.iaedp.com
A membership organization for professionals; provides certification, education, local chapters, a newsletter, a monthly bulletin, and an annual symposium.

NATIONAL EATING DISORDERS ORGANIZATION
6655 S. Yale Ave.
Tulsa, OK 74136
(918) 481-4044
www.laureate.com
Focuses on prevention, education, research, and treatment referrals; distributes information and a newsletter, and holds an annual conference.

OVEREATERS ANONYMOUS HEADQUARTERS
World Services Office
P.O. Box 44020
Rio Rancho, NM 87174-4020
(505) 891-2664
www.overeatersanonymous.org
A 12-step self-help fellowship. Free local meetings are listed in the telephone pages under Overeaters Anonymous.

NATIONAL CENTER for OVERCOMING OVEREATING
315 W. 86th St. #17B
New York, NY 10024
(212) 875-0442
An educational and training organization dedicated to ending body hatred and dieting. Offices in New York, New England, Chicago, Houston and Atlanta.

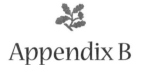

Appendix B

Support Groups

Begin from Within
3272 California St.
San Francisco, CA 94118
(415) 563-0282
www.jfcs.org/bfw.html
Originally developed by the authors of *The Don't Diet, Live-It Workbook,* this program is sponsored by Jewish Family and Children's Services of San Francisco, the Peninsula, Marin and Sonoma Counties. Groups are led by professional therapists who have recovered from eating disorders as well.

Breaking Free
Box 2852
Santa Cruz, CA. 95063
(831) 685-8601
Geneen Roth leads Breaking Free Workshops around the country. These workshops generate support groups that are self-led by workshop participants. The Breaking Free office can help you find a support group or a therapist in your area.

InnerSolutions
5905 Soquel Dr. #650
Soquel, CA 95073
(831) 476-7500
www.innersolutions.net

The authors of *The Don't Diet, Live-It Workbook* co-lead 16-week and ongoing support groups using this workbook as a guide.

Overeaters Anonymous
6075 Zenith Court
Rio Rancho, NM 87124
(505) 891-2664
www.overeatersanonymous.org
This is a free, 12-Step support group with meetings all over the country. There are no official "leaders," but meetings are "led" by volunteers who are members themselves.

Overcoming Overeating
315 W. 86th St. #17B
New York, NY 10024
(212) 875-0442
www.overeatersanonymous.org
Overcoming Overeating offers groups and workshops for people who are interested in the approach laid out in their books: *Overcoming Overeating* and *When Women Stop Hating Their Bodies* by Jane Hirschmann and Carol Muntner.

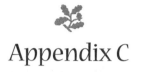

Appendix C

Web Sites

InnerSolutions
www.innersolutions.net
Loving, non-diet approach to healing food, weight and body image issues.

Gürze Books
www.gurze.com
Eating disorders resources and links to other sites.

Something Fishy
www.something-fishy.com
Huge web site with resources for eating disorders.

Geneen Roth
www.geneenroth.com
Pioneered the non-diet approach, leads workshops around the country.

Overcoming Overeating
www.overcomingovereating.com
Campaign to end body hatred; also has books and offers yearly spa or cruise retreats.

Begin from Within
www.jfcs.org/bfw.html
Workshops and therapy groups in Northern California.

Overeaters Anonymous E-mail group
www.hiwaay.net/recovery/

Eating Disorders-Food Addiction Resources
http://www.jps.net/Sunflake/ED.htm

Appendix D

Recommended Reading & Tapes

Books

(Most of these books and many others are available from the *Gürze Eating Disorder Resource Catalogue*. P.O. Box 2238, Carlsbad, CA 92018. Call (800)756-7533 for a free catalog.)

Brown, Stephanie. *Treating the Alcoholic: A Developmental Model of Recovery* John Wiley & Sons Inc., NY 1985. Describes in detail the developmental phases of the addiction recovery process.

Bullitt-Jonas, Margaret. *Holy Hunger: A Memoir of Desire* Random House 1999. A beautifully written true story of the author's journey from the depths of an eating disorder to a spiritually uplifting recovery.

Fodor, Viola. *Desperately Seeking Self: An Inner Guidebook for People with Eating Problems.* Gürze Books, Carlsbad, CA 1997. A lovely book that discusses the important relationship between hunger for food and the need for spiritual connection.

Goodman, Laura. *Is Your Child Dying to be Thin?* Dorrance Publishing Co., Pittsburgh, PA 1992. A workbook for parents and family members on eating disorders.

Hall, Lindsey. *Full Lives: Women Who Have Freed Themselves from Food and Weight Obsession* Gürze Books, Carlsbad, CA 1993. Inspirational accounts of their personal recovery process by best-selling authors.

Hirschmann, Jane and Zaphiropolous, Lela. *Preventing Childhood Eating Problems* Gürze Books, Carlsbad, CA 1993. An insightful book to help both parents and children make peace with food.

Hirschmann, Jane and Munter, Carol. *When Women Stop Hating Their Bodies: Freeing Yourself from Food and Weight Obsession* Ballantine Books, NY 1995. A provocative book to help women redefine themselves and put an end to food deprivation and body hatred.

Johnson, Carol. *Self-Esteem Comes in All Sizes: How to be Happy and Healthy at Your Natural Weight* Doubleday Books, New York, NY 1995. A loving and educational book that is particularly helpful for women with large bodies.

Johnston, Joni. *Appearance Obsession: Learning to Love the Way You Look* Health Communications, Inc. Deerfield Beach, FL 1994. A thorough book addressing the relationship between self-esteem and appearance obsession, with suggestions for becoming more comfortable in one's body.

Louden, Jennifer. *Women's Comfort Book* Harper Books, San Francisco, CA 1992. Encyclopedia of ideas for self-care and nurturance. Also has Couples Comfort Book.

Normandy, Carol; Roark, Lauralee. *It's Not About Food* Grosset-Putnam 1998. These recovering authors share their own experiences and those of their clients in healing from eating disorders. Also includes internal exercises for the reader to do.

Roth, Geneen. *Feeding the Hungry Heart* Robb's Merrill, Indianapolis, 1982. A very readable and graphic description of the experience of bingeing and the pain of compulsive eating.

Roth, Geneen. *When Food is Love* Dutton, New York, 1991. Explores the connection between eating and intimacy.

Roth, Geneen *When You Eat at the Refrigerator, Pull up a Chair* Hyperion, NY 1998. Using humor, personal experience and profound honesty, this easy-to-read book teaches the reader the many essential and varied components of healing from emotional eating and body hatred.

Siegel, M.; Brisman, J.; Weinshel, M. *Surviving an Eating Disorder: Strategies for Families and Friends* HarperPerrenial, San Francisco, CA 1988. An excellent book for parents with many real-life examples.

Waterhouse, Debra. *Like Mother, Like Daughter: How Women are Influenced by Their Mothers' Relationship with Food—and How to Break the Pattern*. Hyperion, New York 1997. Explains the relationship between our dieting culture and the prevalence of eating disorders. Excellent book with tips on understanding and healing your relationship with food and guiding your daughters.

Magazines

MODE Magazine: Style Beyond Size
22 E. 49th St.
New York, NY 10017
(888) 610-6633
modemag@aol.com
A wonderful magazine that uses models of varied sizes, particularly focusing on sizes 12, 14 and 16. This magazine focuses on beauty and fashion and self-acceptance regardless of size. Also available: MODE for Young Girls.

Radiance: The Magazine for Large Women
P.O. Box 30246
Oakland, CA. 94604
(510) 482-0680
www.radiancemagazine.com

An upbeat, positive, colorful, empowering, glossy quarterly magazine in its second decade of print. They support readers in living proud, full, active lives filled with self love and self respect.

Tapes

Love Your Body by Louise Hay
3029 Wilshire Blvd.
Santa Monica CA. 90404
(800) 654-5126
Positive affirmations for learning to love your body, based on the book by the same name. Hearing affirmations on a continual basis can bring positive changes to your self image.

InnerJourneys by InnerSolutions
5905 Soquel Dr. #650
Soquel, CA. 95073
(831) 476-7500
The authors of *The Don't Diet Live-It Workbook* guide the listener through three separate "journeys" or visualizations designed to help heal food, weight and body image issues.

Transforming Body Image by Marcia Germaine Hutchinson, Ed.D
Gürze Books
P.O. Box 2238
Carlsbad, CA. 92018
(800) 756-7533
This tape offers women several exercises to aid in the process of healing your body image. Based on book of the same name.

Overweight Workshop I by Patricia Sun
P.O. Box 7065
Berkeley, CA. 94707
(510) 532-4160
A powerful workshop that focuses on the difference between our logical and intuitive minds. This understanding helps in the transition from diet mentality to a Live-It.

Breaking Free: The Workshop by Geneen Roth
Breaking Free
Box 2852
Santa Cruz, CA. 95063
(831) 685-8601
Cassette series of Geneen Roth's workshops in which she conducts powerful exercises and visualizations for anyone who is trying to heal from the diet/binge cycle.

Appendix E

Leading Live-It® Groups

If you are a psychotherapist or a mental health professional, you may be interested in starting a Live-It® Group in your area. Utilizing *The Don't Diet, Live-It Workbook*, in conjunction with peer support and professionally facilitated groups, creates the most powerful combination for producing change in clients with food, weight, and body image issues. This section is written for those who are interested in knowing more about how we run our Live-It Groups. In the first part, we will explain the structure we utilize in our groups; in the second part, we will describe typical presenting issues and some of the responses and techniques we use to handle them.

As you probably know, people with food, weight, and body issues tend to isolate themselves and often have difficulty turning to people (rather than food) for support. In Live-It groups, clients can learn how to develop healthy, honest, and supportive relationships. Eventually, as members learn to trust each other and take care of themselves, they become a support system for each other throughout the week, rather than just during group time. Additionally, clients working with *The Don't Diet, Live-It Workbook*, find that a support group can provide a safe environment in which to deal with the feelings that arise as they proceed through the workbook.

Because groups that deal with food, weight, and body image inevitably lead into deeper issues, we believe that these groups must be led by a licensed mental health professional. We have also found that professionals who have themselves fought and won their own battles with weight and body image are most naturally sympathetic to and understanding of the long and arduous process of recovery. If this is your situation, your own experience is an asset that provides hope and reassurance during your clients' recovery process. We also believe that it is important for you to live by the principles you teach, and that you utilize your own support system, such as supervision or consultation, when you are dealing with difficult group or personal issues. (If you feel that you are in need of additional assistance, InnerSolutions offers telephone consultations to support you in your work with individuals and groups dealing with food, weight and body image issues.)

Live-It Groups

Length and frequency of meetings:
Our groups last 90 minutes and are held once a week for 15 weeks. This allows one week for each chapter in the workbook. We limit our groups to a maximum of eight people.

Screening:
We have separate groups for adults and for teens. We do, however, include all forms, styles, and degrees of weight and body issues in our groups, because though the symptoms are different, the issues and the solutions are similar. All members must be medically stable, or we refer them to a doctor or inpatient treatment. If we determine that a person seems particularly needy or fearful of a group setting, we may arrange for some individual therapy sessions before the group begins. It can sometimes be difficult to immediately assess a personality disorder. However, if we sense that someone may be disruptive to a group, we refer them to individual therapy instead. Some questions to consider are:

> Is the client on medication of any sort?
> Have they ever been hospitalized?
> Is there any history of suicide attempts?
> Do they have any other addictions or obsessions?
> Are they currently or have they ever been in any type of therapy?

Though we do not rule out people who answer yes to any of these questions, we may require release forms of information, or referrals to additional treatment (psychiatrists, A.A., individual or couples therapy) in order for them to attend the group.

Before the first meeting:
When members register for the group, they buy a copy of *The Don't Diet, Live-It Workbook*. We ask them to read the Introduction before the first group and to write a brief history of their lives, including their food and weight issues. There are two examples of this on pages one through four of the *Workbook* Introduction. We request that they bring their written histories to the first group.

First group structure:

Here is a list of activities we suggest for your first group, followed by detailed explanations of each activity:

• Hand out Group Guidelines and Participation Agreements.
• Get to know members' names through an icebreaker activity.
• Address questions regarding handouts.
• Collect signed Participation Agreements and review pertinent logistics.
• Teach and do "check-ins."
• Group Introductions.
• Begin Personal Histories.

The following are detailed explanations of how we conduct the above activities:

First, we hand out the Group Guidelines and Participation Agreements. (See samples on page 255) We do this while people are arriving so that group members have something to do while they are waiting for the group to begin.

Then, we get to know group members' names through a fun icebreaker. One "name game" we use is to have clients say their first names followed by something they like which begins with the first letter of their names. For example: "I'm Alice and I like Animals." It can also be fun to bring in a variety of household items or toys and have the clients pick one that most represents them, then introduce the item to the group as if they were introducing themselves.

Next, we address questions about the handouts. We especially review confidentiality and post-group feelings. We explain that confidentiality means that everything said in the group stays within the group, and that no one will reveal the identity of group members to anyone outside of the group. We make sure group members read the limits to confidentiality that are listed on the Participation Agreement handout. We also tell members that if we see them in public, we will not acknowledge them in any way other than, perhaps, a loving smile.

We remind group members that when working on vulnerable issues such as food and body image, many feelings will come up after and between groups. We call these "post-group feelings." We suggest that members keep a journal in which they can record their feelings, or that they make phone contact with other group members in between groups, if that is agreed upon within the group. We encourage them to attend self-help, non-dieting support groups, such as Overeaters Anonymous, Breaking Free, or Overcoming Overeating, and to utilize their individual psychotherapist, if they have one.

We then collect the signed Participation Agreements. We review group dates, payment procedures, and any other pertinent logistics. We also request that if a member cannot attend a session, she will let at least one other person in the group know. We explain that this keeps the group feeling cohesive, even when someone cannot attend. We also remind them that they are expected to pay for each group in their 16-week commitment whether they attend or not. This encourages attendance, which is especially needed when a member is ambivalent about coming to group.

At this point we shift the focus. We teach and do "check-ins" which formally begins the actual group process. We ask each member to say three words to describe what they are feeling in that moment. For example, "I am feeling scared, anxious and excited," or "I am feeling nervous, sad and angry." We emphasize that there are no right or wrong feelings; they can even feel sad and happy at the same time. We convey acceptance by not commenting on or judging anyone's feelings. This helps members see that all their feelings are welcome. There are a few exceptions to this: if a group member is numb or disconnected from her feelings, we may encourage her to take a deep breath and see if she can connect, or even guess what she might be feeling. We also educate the members that "fat" is not a feeling, and we encourage them to look further or get more specific if they use "fat" to describe their feelings. The same applies if they describe their feelings as "good" or "bad."

As group leaders, we do not participate in the check-in, and if the group questions that, we let them know we get our support elsewhere and are there to facilitate, not participate in, the group.

For Group Introductions each participant answers the following three questions aloud:

1. What brought you to this group?
2. What are your fears about being in this group?
3. What are your hopes about being in this group?

After each person has completed the Introductions, we ask for volunteers to read their Personal Histories. We are careful to be supportive of different manners in which the members complete this. We do, however, encourage those who have written their history to read it, and we invite those who have not yet written theirs to do so during the week. We do not interrupt the telling of a members' history unless they do not seem present. If this is the case, we encourage them to slow down, breathe, or share any fears preventing them from being present. Following the history, we ask the participant to do a "check-in" and see if she would like feedback from the other group members. Feedback helps the person who told her story to feel connected to the group, and it helps the members recognize and verbalize the ways in which they relate to one another. In order to keep the feedback responsible and productive, we encourage members to stick to the following three guidelines:

a. what they related to in the story they just heard
b. what touched them about the story or how it was told
c. what feelings they felt while listening to the story

We remind members to speak from the first person "I" as much as possible, and to keep the feedback brief so that the focus remains on the storyteller.

At the end of the first group, and each of the following groups, we remind members to read the next chapter in *The Don't Diet, Live-It Workbook* and to bring their Journey writings to next week's group. Though we sometimes do not get to the chapters in much detail until after the histories are complete, we encourage participants to complete the reading and the exercises. Usually by the third or fourth week, all participants have read their histories and there is time to go over the chapters in more detail.

Ongoing group structure:

Once all the members have finished their histories, we begin each week with the check-in as described above, then allow time for members to either read what they wrote in their workbooks, or talk about that particular chapter and how it relates to their lives, their struggles with food and weight, or their recoveries. From here, we follow the group process and respond to whatever issues emerge, sometimes focusing on an individual, sometimes addressing the group as a whole. We believe that experiential work is critical in helping clients identify and express feelings, so we utilize gestalt and process work in all our groups. (In the second half of this section, we go into more detail about the typical issues that come up in the groups and how we work with them.)

After the second week of group, we encourage members to create an optional phone list (with times they are most likely to be available) so they can call each other during the week. Throughout the group sessions, we emphasize the importance of making contact with each other between groups in order to create and utilize a daily support system that can replace their self-destructive reliance on food.

We remind members that the feelings they have been stuffing down are likely to start coming to the surface as they progress on their Journeys. We encourage them to begin building a support system by making calls to each other between groups. We suggest that they initially view these calls as "practice calls" and make one or two calls per week to get used to the idea of reaching out. We remind them that if they don't practice making connections during less stressful times, it will be even more difficult to reach out when they really need help, like just before a binge. We teach members that a support system means that no one person is responsible for anyone in the group. On a hard day, a member can call several people for support. We remind them that support is not about saving or fixing someone, or solving their problems, it is about being there, listening, and experiencing the ebbs and flows of recovery together. We also emphasize the importance of letting each other know when one doesn't feel like talking or is unavailable for support. We remind them that not only are there always others who can be called, but also that their honesty can make them more trustworthy and strengthen their relationships. In addition to helping members set up and utilize a support system, we help them, in the group, to identify and "unstuff" the emotions that contribute to their food and weight issues. This is the ongoing work of the group which involves maintaining group safety, and gently and lovingly guiding members toward their feelings.

Following are our goals for clients completing their first 16-week group:

• a thorough understanding of why diets do not work
• a basic understanding of the emotions and personal issues that contribute to their food and weight problems
• an understanding of the importance of breaking isolation and receiving support around their personal issues
• an awareness of the relationship between their feelings and their over- or undereating and body hatred

- identification of who in their lives are "safe people" and who are not
- beginning ability to use safe people for support
- beginning ability to distinguish between physical and emotional hunger
- ability to "check-in" and identify feelings, as distinguished from thoughts
- beginning ability to feel and express emotions
- recognition of their internal critical voice
- awareness of the role their critical voice plays in their food and weight issues
- understanding that their food and weight issues are not caused by weakness or lack of willpower
- comprehension of recovery as a process, and awareness of where they are in that process

Last group:

Stressing the importance of closure, we begin reminding the group of the last session about a month before its arrival. We use the last group meeting to say good-bye. We invite each group member to answer the following three questions aloud:

1. What did you get from your participation in this group?
2. What didn't you get that you wish you had?
3. How do you plan to continue your recovery process?

We also encourage members to share important memories from the group as well as things they have appreciated about other participants. Then each member takes a turn saying "Good-bye" to the group, breathing, and feeling the feelings that go with this ending. After all the good-byes are said, we end the group.

Journey Two, Three, and Four Groups:

At some point in the last month of the group, we start discussing options for upcoming groups so that those who want to continue with Journey Two, Three, or Four can register. Then we open registrations to the community and fill the remaining spaces with new members.

When a new member joins the group, she is asked to read the *Workbook* Introduction prior to group and to start working on her food and weight history. She then reads the same chapters in the workbook as the other group members, but answers Journey One questions, while the other members work on the questions from either Journeys Two, Three, or Four.

Common Problems Encountered by Group Leaders

Psychotherapists frequently consult with us about group dynamics and problematic situations. The following are some common problems and our methods of handling them. Because most people who suffer from weight and body image issues are very disconnected from their feelings, we put an emphasis on experiential work in our groups. We strive to help the clients connect with their feelings in the group, rather than talk or intellectualize about their feelings. Many of the interventions below reflect this emphasis. We strongly recommend that you get training in experiential work if you have not already done so.

1. When asked what she is feeling, a client says "numb."

We tell our clients that "numb" is not a feeling, but a state of being disconnected from feelings.

• We ask the client to "guess" what she might be feeling if she wasn't numb.

• We ask if she would like help, and we invite the group members to guess, based on the nonverbal cues they are seeing or what they might be feeling if they were in this person's situation.

• We also might suggest that the client describe the physical feelings she currently notices in her body. This helps her to begin learning how to connect with her emotions.

• We might give her a list of feelings and invite her to pick all those she might be experiencing.

• We might tell her it is fine to be numb right now, that we have great respect for protective defenses. We ask her to take a few deep breaths and to look around the room and notice the support and love that is coming from the other group members. (This may connect her to her feelings.)

2. The client says her only problem is her weight.

When a client is insistent that she only wants to talk about food or weight, we view that as the doorway we must go through to find out more about her.

• We ask her to tell us all about her weight problem. We help her to access and experience her emotions while doing so. We do this by noting or inquiring about her feelings while she is talking. If tears arise, we encourage her to welcome the tears rather than to stuff them back down. If she seems angry, we encourage her to show it and let us see just how angry she is.

• We might ask her to put her weight in an empty chair and say whatever she wants to it. We will then notice what she does with her feelings, i.e. refuse to express them, smile while verbalizing anger, or dissociate. We work with her on expressing her feelings congruently.

• We might ask her to go around the room and tell each group member a problem she has with her weight and then go around the room again and tell each group member a non weight-related thing she struggles with in her life.

• We might hand her a pillow and say, "This is your weight. What do you want to do or say to it right now?" We then encourage her to express her feelings in any way that comes to her. (She may want to beat it up, yell at it, or ask it some questions.) We may make suggestions, if needed, such as, "If this seems true to you, tell your weight: I'll only be happy when you change." If this creates awareness of the irony, and the client says, "That's not true," we then say, "Tell your weight what is true." At some point in the process we may also ask her to take on the voice of the weight and let it respond to what she has been saying.

3. This client feels she has so many problems, she doesn't know where to begin.

Many clients go through a phase of being overwhelmed when they first begin to have access to suppressed feelings. We reassure them that this is a normal part of The Transition Stage of Recovery (see pg. 17). If, however, the client seems too needy for the group on an ongoing basis, we will refer her to individual therapy sessions in addition to the group and encourage her to attend self-help groups as well. If this is not sufficient in meeting her needs, we will encourage her to do intensive individual therapy rather than participate in the group at this time. Here are some ways we deal with a group member who has a number of different problematic issues:

• We ask the client to sit quietly for a minute and ask her heart, or intuition, what to focus on first.

• We suggest that the client focus on the current moment and explore all the feelings and body sensations of which she is presently aware.

• We ask the client to list all her problems, including what feelings she has about each one. We may ask her to prioritize the list, or to come up with one "action step" for addressing each issue.

• We might hand the client a basket of blocks and ask her to pick one for every problem in her life and tell us what each one is. When she is done, we ask her what she would like to do with the pile. We then follow her process from there, encouraging her to do what she wants with the pile, then checking in with her on the feelings that arise.

4. The client says she's starting a new diet.

Although we know that diets don't work, we continue to support clients who are on diets and recognize that they may not have finished learning whatever they need to learn from dieting.

• We encourage them to continue coming to group to maintain their support system.

• We may share some of our personal histories with dieting and let them know that we remember thinking that a diet would solve our problems too.

• We lovingly and non-judgmentally ask them about their dieting history. We then ask what they think will make this attempt different.

• We encourage them to identify and explore the feelings that precipitated their decision to go on a diet. We discuss the needs they have and question whether or not the diet addresses those needs. We encourage the client to discover alternate ways of meeting those needs, whether she decides to stay on the diet or not.

• We put a pillow, representing the diet, on a chair across from the client and ask the client to tell the diet her hopes and her fears.

5. One client goes on and on talking about herself without disclosing her feelings, yet says she doesn't have a problem expressing her feelings.

There is a difference between talking about emotions and actually feeling and expressing them. People with food and weight issues often intellectualize, rather than feel, their emotions. This keeps them from finding resolution and moving on. As group leaders we try to help members learn how to connect with their feelings rather than just talk about them.

• We encourage the client to go around the room and tell each group member, in one sentence, what she is feeling. We then ask her what the experience was like and how it was different from the way she normally expresses feelings.

• We tell the client that sometimes we start to disconnect while she is talking. We ask her if, when that happens, we can interrupt and ask her what she is feeling at the time and whether or not she is connected to her feelings.

• We encourage her to notice when her talking is superficial and when it feels intimate. We help her explore and define the difference between the two. We carefully suggest that some people avoid feelings by not talking, while others avoid them by over talking.

• We let the client know that although what she says is interesting and important, her recovery will benefit by her learning how to slow down and be quiet at times.

• We ask if she is open to group feedback as to how they see her expressing or avoiding feelings.

• We ask her what she does think she has problems with, and what kind of support she would like from the group.

• We ask if she is willing to try an experiment. If so, we invite her to be silent for 1-2 minutes. We ask her to simply breathe and notice what it is like to receive attention from the group without having to do or say anything. Then we ask her to describe what it was like and what feelings she noticed.

6. A client says she's been bingeing all week and her eating has gotten worse, not better, since joining the group.

Depending on our assessment of the severity of her situation, we may refer her to a psychiatrist for medication, to individual therapy, or to a self-help group.

• We explore her current support system and the degree to which she is using it. We encourage her to make a commitment to the group to increase the amount of support she receives. For example, we may ask her to commit to the group that she will call at least two members during the week and will discuss with them whatever she is feeling at the time.

• We normalize her bingeing experience by educating her about the process of recovery. We explain that the group, or something else in her life, is probably bringing up feelings, and that her response to having uncomfortable feelings has always been to eat. We assure her that most people feel worse before they get better because they are just learning to feel again, after years of being disconnected from their feelings.

• We explain that every binge has a reason and a voice. We ask her what her bingeing is trying to tell her.

• We ask her to imagine herself during a recent binge, and to become an observer of it. (Perhaps she was sitting in front of the TV, or standing at her kitchen counter.) We invite her to speak to the binger, to ask her what she is needing, and then listen to the response.

• We might invite the client to tell each group member one situation or emotion she might have been trying to forget or soothe by eating.

• We remind her that in the early stages of recovery, people need an enormous amount of support. We ask her to come up with one way she could reach out to a person rather than to food. Sometimes we self-disclose some of the struggles we experienced when learning how to reach out to others and the ways in which support from them has helped us.

• We remind her that people who are just beginning the process of recovery don't suddenly stop bingeing and cease to ever binge again. We explain that bingeing is a coping style that she has used for a long time, and that as she learns other, more effective, coping strategies, she will have fewer desires to binge.

As You Begin Creating a Safe Place...

It is profoundly satisfying to help people escape the prison of food, weight and body obsession. We hope that this section of The Don't Diet, Live-It Workbook can assist you in carrying out the mission to end body hatred and compulsive eating. We know that there is a way out, and that way is through the feelings. As you begin to create a safe place for people to feel their way through recovery, we hope that you remember to create and use your own safe places. We, at InnerSolutions, offer phone consultations, so feel free to contact us and inquire about our rates if you would like our support. Best wishes to you in guiding others on their Journeys!

Please remember: Live-It® is a trademark of InnerSolutions™. InnerSolutions' trademarks my not be used publicly without the express permission of InnerSolutions. Fair use of InnerSolutions' trademarks in advertising and promotion of InnerSolutions' products requires proper acknowledgment. InnerSolutions does not endorse or recommend any specific facilitators who use The Don't Diet Live-It Workbook in their groups. Participants in groups which use The Don't Diet, Live-It Workbook have the obligation to investigate the facilitators of these groups independently; and participants have no relationship with InnerSolutions by virtue of participating in a group run by other providers using The Don't Diet, Live-It Workbook.

Group Guidelines (example)

1. Be honest with your feelings and thoughts.

2. Be respectful of yourself and others.

3. Respect the confidentiality of group members.

4. Speak from the first person "I" as much as possible.

5. Be aware of how people in the group remind you of others.

6. Be aware of how feelings in the group remind you of past situations.

7. Expect periods of silence.

8. Come sober to group.

9. Expect post-group feelings.

10. Inform someone in the group if you are unable to make it to a session.

Participation and Confidentiality Agreement (example)

Food, Weight and Body Image Group Participation Agreement

Please read and sign:

I understand that I am making a commitment to attend 16 weeks of group therapy. Sessions will be paid for weekly, one week in advance, including missed sessions. The group cost is $____ per week. I understand that while I am a member of the group, I will be expected to pay each week, whether I am able to attend group or not.

I will make every effort to arrive on time and if I am unable to attend a group I will let someone in the group know.

I will maintain the confidentiality of the other group members and I will not reveal any personal information about anyone in the group.

I understand that the exceptions to therapist/client confidentiality include:
1) intention or knowledge of harm to self or others
2) any knowledge of physical or sexual abuse of a minor or dependent adult
3) a court order

Client Signature:_____   Date: _____

About the Authors

Andrea Wachter is a licensed marriage and family therapist who specializes in the healing of food, weight, and body image issues. She lectures and writes extensively on these subjects and has appeared on several radio and television shows. Andrea received her Master's degree from the University of San Francisco. Currently, she is in private practice in Soquel, California where she works with adults, adolescents, families, and groups.

Marsea Marcus is a licensed marriage and family therapist specializing in the healing of eating disorders, depression, and sexual abuse. She obtained her Master's degree from John F. Kennedy University and is also a trained process therapist. Marsea has worked as a clinician at The Rader Institute and several other inpatient treatment centers for eating disorders and addiction recovery. Recently she was Program Coordinator for Begin from Within, Center for Resolving Food and Weight Issues and presently she has a private practice in Northern California.

Both of the authors are cofounders of InnerSolutions, a counseling service dedicated to helping people heal from food, weight, and body image issues. In addition to individual, family, and group counseling, they offer interventions for families dealing with members who have severe eating disorders. They also conduct supervision and training for other therapists and counseling agencies. Marcus and LoBue are both inspirational speakers who bring expertise, humor, and stories of personal recovery to their audiences. Their motivation comes from having successfully dealt with these issues in their own lives.

The authors, who also offer tapes, can be contacted at: InnerSolutions; 5905 Soquel Dr. #650; Soquel, CA 95073; (831) 476-7500; www.innersolutions.net.

To Order Books or FREE Catalogue

Copies of the *Don't Diet, Live-It! Workbook* are available at bookstores or directly from Gürze Books, who offers quantity discounts.

The *Gürze Eating Disorders Resource Catalogue* has more than 130 books and tapes on eating disorders and related topics. It is a valuable resource that is handed out by health care professionals throughout the world.

Gürze Books; PO Box 2238; Carlsbad, CA 92018
(800) 756-7533 • www.gurze.com